388 Great Hairstyles

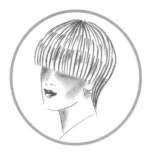

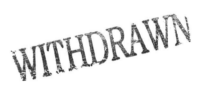

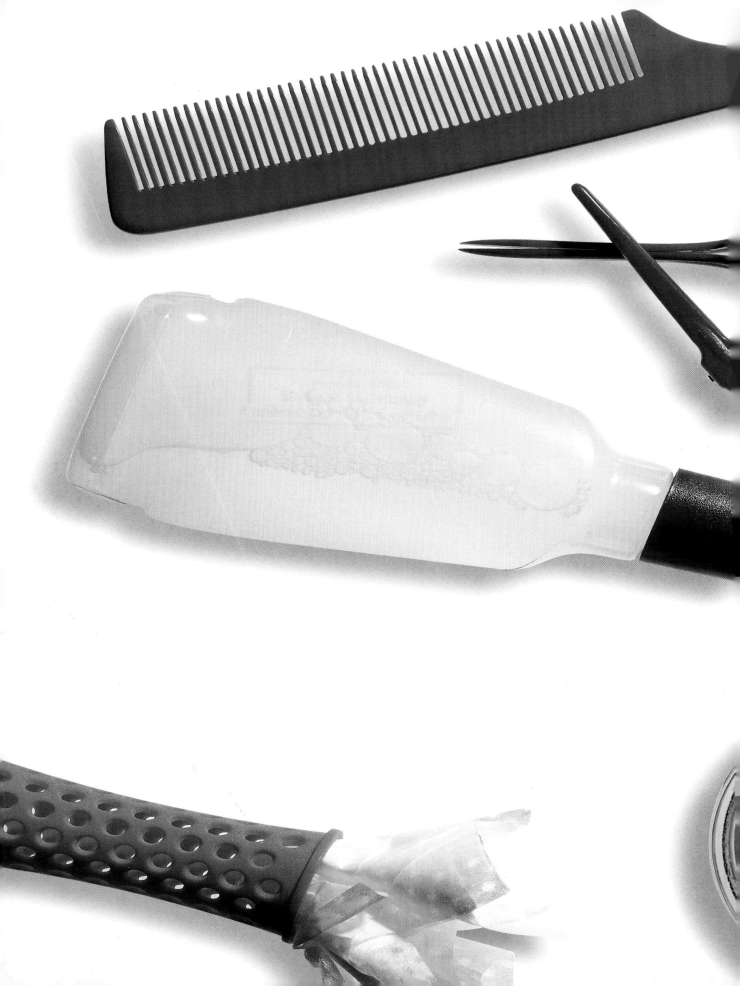

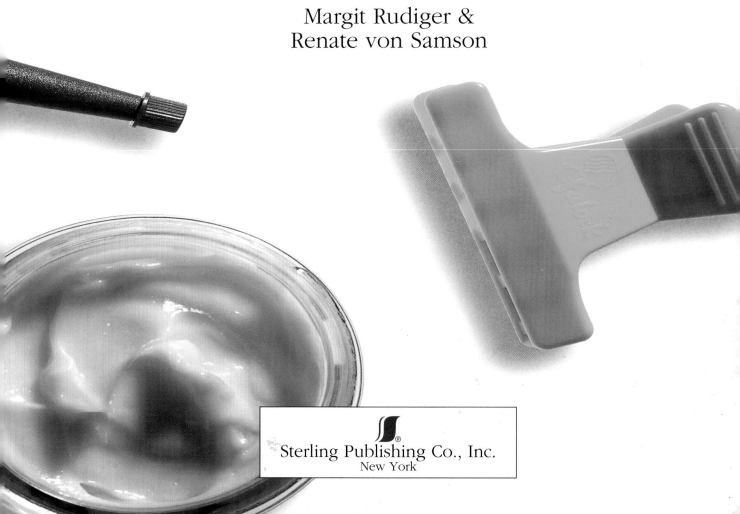

388 *Great*
Hairstyles

Margit Rudiger &
Renate von Samson

Sterling Publishing Co., Inc.
New York

Every effort has been made to ensure that all the information in the book is accurate. However, due to differing conditions, tools and individual skills, neither the publisher nor the authors can be responsible for any injuries, losses, and other damages which may result from the information in this book.

Drawings by Chris Menke
English translation by Elisabeth Reinersmann; English translation edited by Isabel Stein

Library of Congress Cataloging-in-Publication Data
Rüdiger, Margit.
        [388 Frisuren für jede Länge, für jeden Typ, für jede Gelegenheit. English]
        388 great hairstyles / Margit Rudiger & Renate von Samson.
            p. cm.
        Includes index.
        ISBN 0-8069-9401-0
        1. Hairdressing. I. Von Samson, Renate. II. Title.
    TT972R7313   1998
        646.7'24—dc21   97-51848
                                                                CIP

10 9 8 7

Published by Sterling Publishing Co., Inc.
387 Park Avenue South, New York, N.Y. 10016
Originally published in Germany under the title *388 Frisuren für jede Länge, für jeden Typ, für jede Gelegenheit* by Margit Rüdiger and Renate von Samson
© 1997 by FALKEN-Verlag GmBH Niedernhausen/Ts., Germany
English translation ©1998 by Sterling Publishing Co.
Distributed in Canada by Sterling Publishing
c/o Canadian Manda Group, One Atlantic Avenue, Suite 105
Toronto, Ontario, Canada M6K 3E7
Distributed in Great Britain by Chrysalis Books
64 Brewery Road, London N7 9NT, England
Distributed in Australia by Capricorn Link (Australia) Pty Ltd.
P.O. Box 704, Windsor, NSW 2756 Australia
Printed in Hong Kong

Sterling ISBN 0–8069–9401–0

When your hair looks good, it makes you feel good. If, like most women, you're busy and on the go all week, you want a style that's easy to wear, simple to do, and one which can be quickly changed to give you a variety of looks.

Here is a collection of hundreds of hairstyles for you to choose from. Starting with 18 basic haircuts, there are a wide variety of styles to suit your mood, style, and the occasion—including sporty, classic, and romantic looks and dressed-up styles for a night out. You'll find advice specifically for your hair length and hair type—whether it is short or long, curly or straight, dry or oily, naturally wavy or permed. A section about face shapes helps you choose styles that will look good on you. And turn to the quick-drying super cuts for fast and painless hair care.

Cutting and styling information and hundreds of photos and drawings show how to achieve a wide range of hairstyles from your basic cut. There's also advice about perming and coloring, and the situation that can be most traumatic: a trip to the hairstylist's. When you go to the salon, take this book in hand to help insure that your trip has a happy ending. If you style your hair at home, keep it by your vanity table; you'll find valuable tips on how to achieve the look you want, while still being kind to your hair.

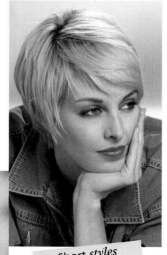

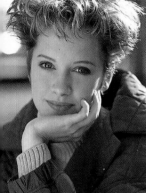

Short full *styles*

Medium *styles*

Short *styles*

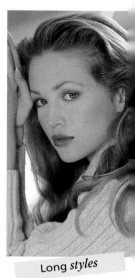

Long *styles*

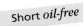

Short *oil-free*

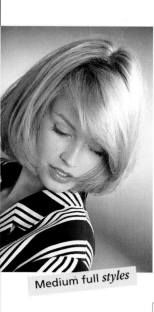

Medium full *styles*

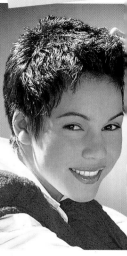

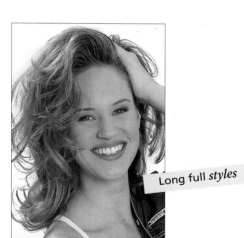

Long full *styles*

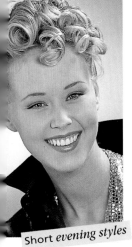
Short *evening styles*

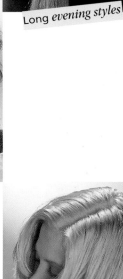
Long *evening styles*

CHAPTER III
Evening styles

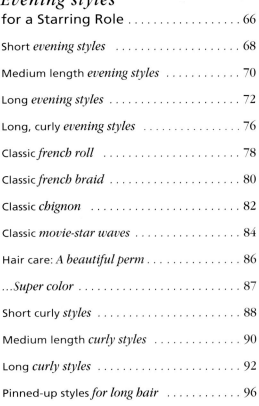
Long *evening styles*

CHAPTER IV
Choose a style Just for You

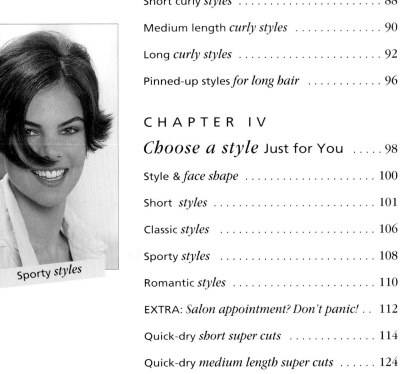
Sporty *styles*

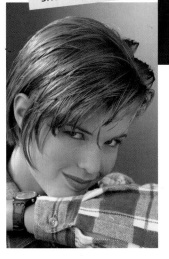
Short *super cuts*

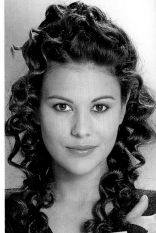
Medium *super cuts*

CHAPTER I

Choices: 18 HAIR

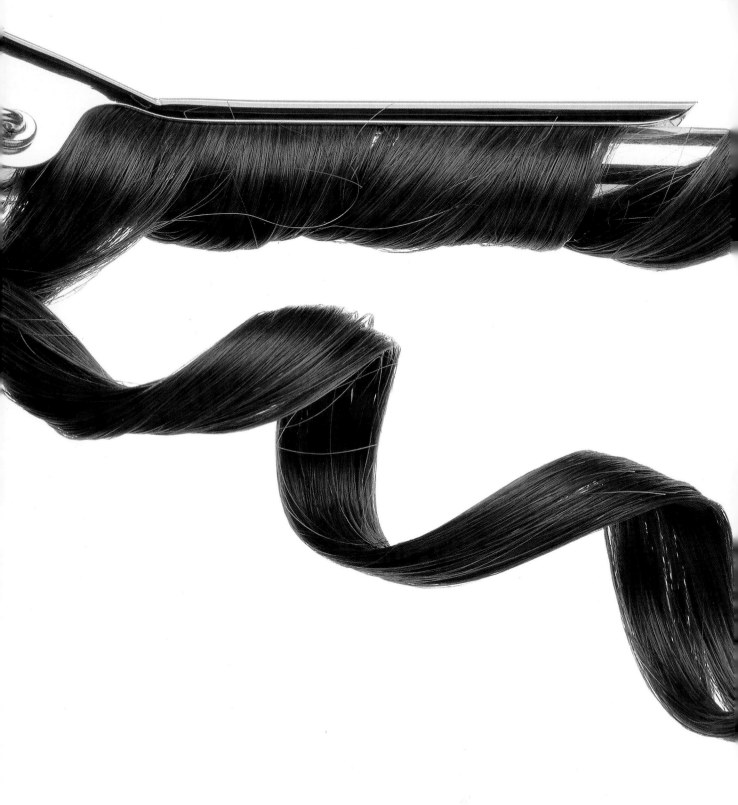

UTS TO PLAY WITH

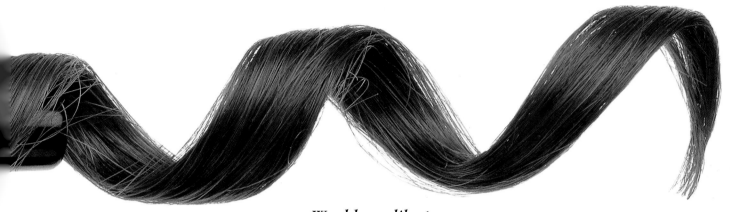

Would you like to
change your hairstyle
without having to go to the
hairstylist's? No problem! Using a few tricks,
the haircuts that we present on the next pages
are easy to change. A drawing of each basic cut
is given, plus the styles you can
make with it.

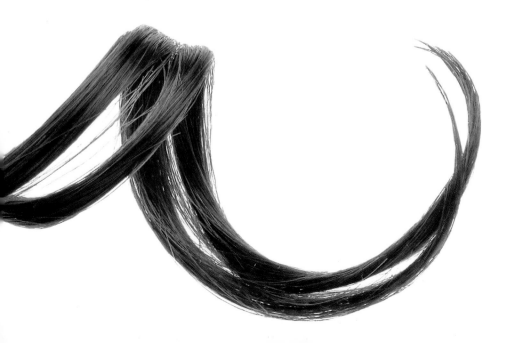

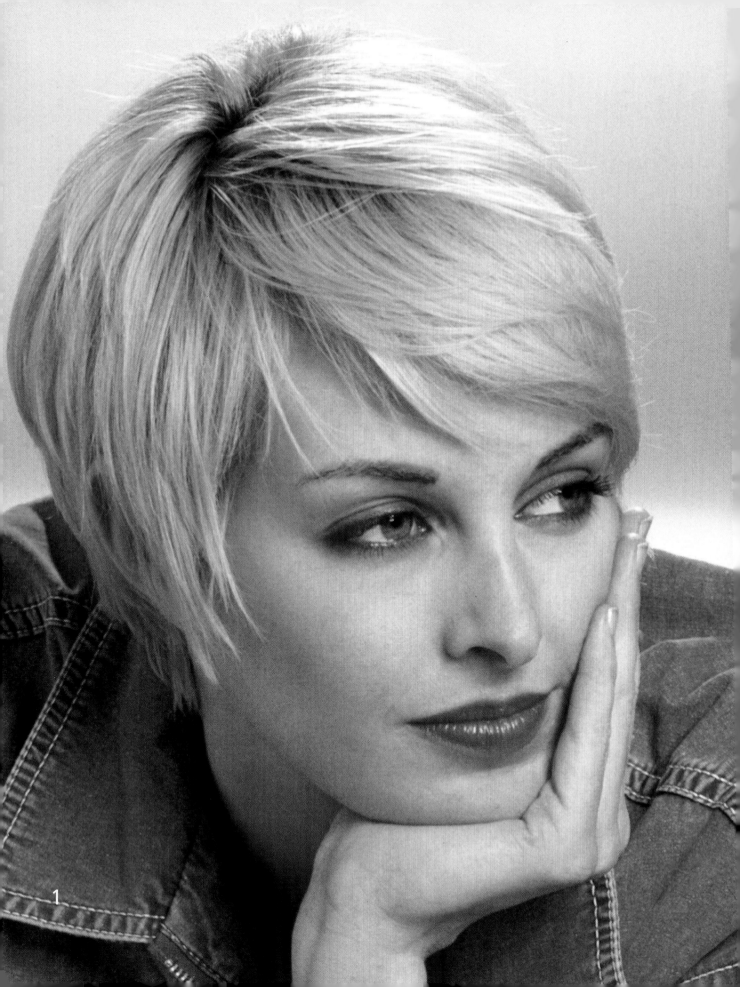

SHORT *styles*

1 *Smooth: When blow-drying, pull one lock at a time slowly over a vent brush. Use a gel wax for the sideburns.* **2** *Stiff bangs: Part hair on the side. With styling gel rubbed on the palms, draw your hands through the bangs from underneath, lifting until hair is off forehead.* **3** *One lock of hair at a time is curled with a curling iron. Use fingers to place curls.* **4** *Bend head down and dry hair, moving dryer back and forth over hair.* Apply hair spray one lock at a time to the ends. **5** *Apply styling liquid to damp hair. Form waves with a comb and the edge of your hand. Secure with clips. Let air-dry naturally or use a diffuser.*

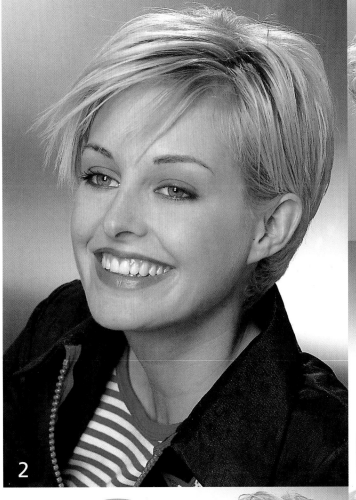

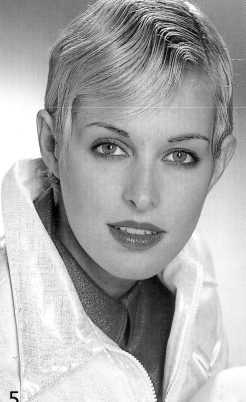

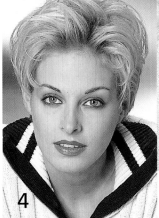

The cut:
Top layer is layered with long bangs and short at the neck. Also works well with fine hair

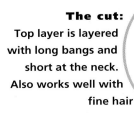

6 *1960s style: Part the hair in the middle; apply styling gel to the left and right of the part to smooth and stiffen each strand. Tease the hair at back of head.* **7** *With the curling iron, gently curl the bangs. Part the hair unevenly and fasten one side with a barrette. Pull the curled bangs into shape on the forehead.* **8** *Tousled look: Massage volumizing mousse into the dry hair; pull each individual lock through a curling iron. Use fingers to create a tousled look.* **9** *Mushroom: After shampooing, blow-dry hair over a round brush towards the front. Apply styling gel to the ends.*

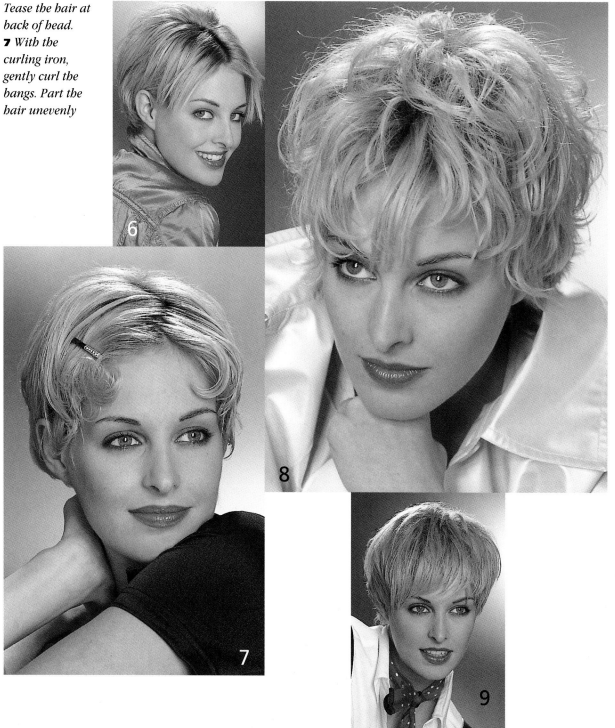

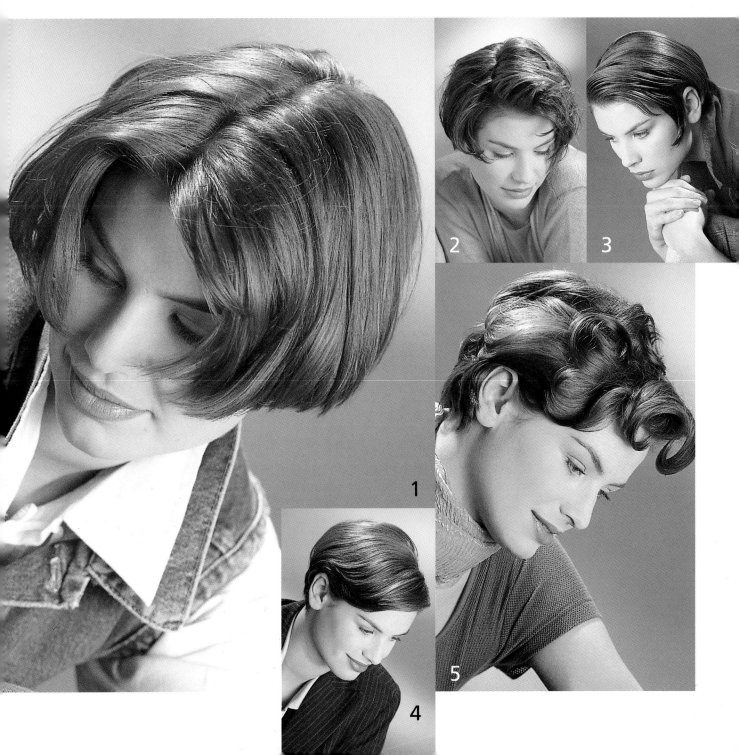

The cut:
A short bob, slightly slanted at the neck. The face contour and the forehead area are slightly layered to give hair more volume and make it easier to style

1 *The rounded look: From the center part out, blow-dry the hair over a round brush to the inside. Apply styling gel and gently massage the hair.* **2** *Shaggy:*

Blow-dry hair one lock at a time over a round brush to give it body. The front is styled with gel wax and blow-dried upwards using a brush. **3** *Close to the head:*

Moisten hair with styling liquid. Part hair low on one side and comb close to the head; sides are curved forward. **4** *Tomboy: Apply styling gel, comb hair back*

into a soft wave behind the ears. **5** *Clip curls: Dampen hair with styling liquid; fasten curls with clips. When dry, hold with hair spray.*

The cut: Mushroom cut, short and layered in back. Starting at the crown, the top layer is layered equally on all sides and in front reaches above the eyebrows

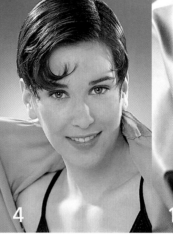

1 *Full:* Starting at the crown, blow-dry hair forward and down around head.
2 *Sporty:* Zigzag flexible comb is pushed into hair above hairline. Hair ends

lightly teased.
3 *Elegant:* Use styling gel; comb close to head; make soft waves with comb and hand. Use hair spray.
4 *Chic:* Apply styling gel and comb; ends are curled at the forehead.

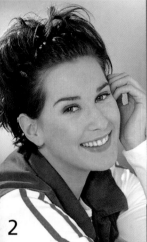

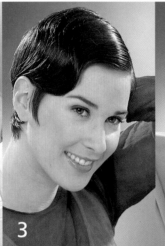

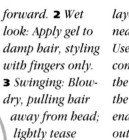

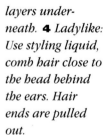

2

3

4

1

The cut: Short, fringed cut, full at the back. Finely layered ends provide volume

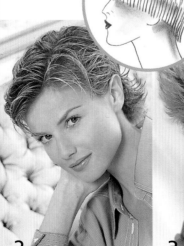

1 *Sporty natural:* Blow-dry hair and with a styling brush, pull hair

forward. **2** *Wet look:* Apply gel to damp hair, styling with fingers only.
3 *Swinging:* Blow-dry, pulling hair away from head; lightly tease

layers underneath. **4** *Ladylike:* Use styling liquid, comb hair close to the head behind the ears. Hair ends are pulled out.

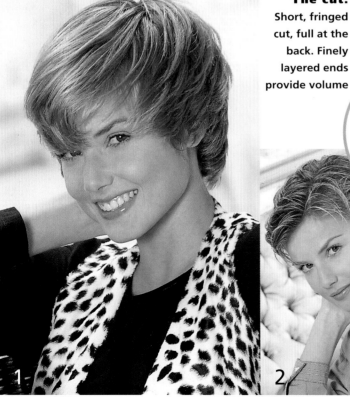

1

2

3

4

The cut:
A full-bodied, heavy top layer, equally long all around, and only slightly layered at the ends. Neck hair short and layered

1 *Fringed: Straighten hair by pulling it through a curling iron. Add styling gel and twist hair between fingers for straggly look.* **2** *Curly: Top layer hair is set on heated curlers. Remove curlers when dry, add gel, and tousle with fingers.* **3** *Fringed: Blow-dry hair forward at an angle towards face.* **4** *Teased: Part hair at an angle. Tease well at back of head, slightly in front. Add styling lacquer to hold.*

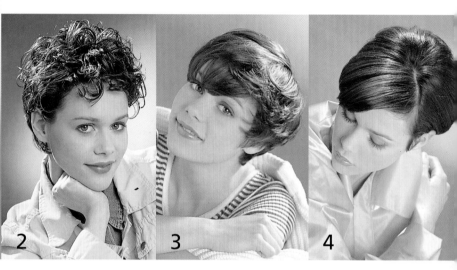

1 2 3 4

1 *With gel: Styling gel or styling liquid is applied to the palm and vigorously rubbed into the hair. Use fingers to comb forward.* **2** *Blow-dried: Starting at the crown, blow-dry hair in individual locks over a brush, pulling to create tension.* **3** *Stand-up bangs: Part hair on the side. Blow-dry hair upwards on the wide side over a small round brush, and apply styling lacquer. Sides are fringed forward.*

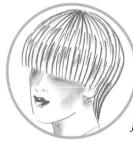

The cut:
Cut hair in short distinct layers; delicate strands frame the face. The neck remains relatively full

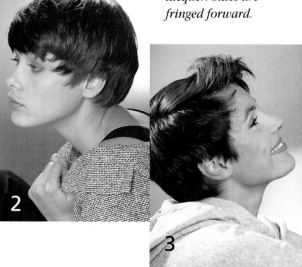

2

3

1

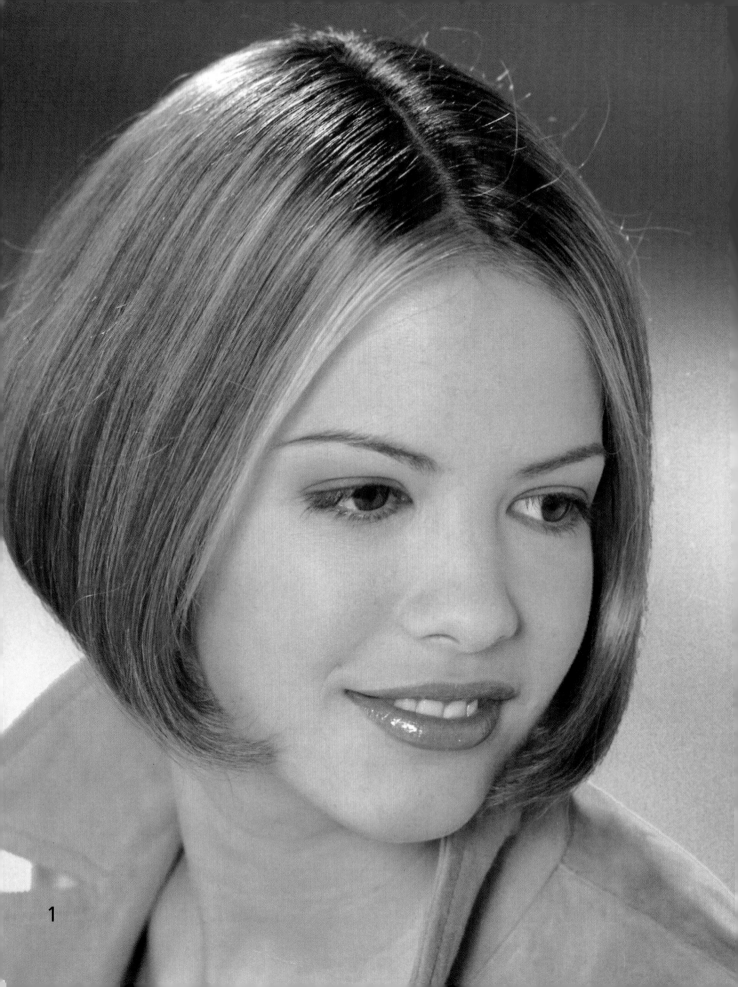

1

MEDIUM LENGTH *styles*

1 *Pageboy with a middle part: Blow-dry hair one lock at a time over a thick round brush, turning hair towards the inside.* **2** *Super curls: Thin locks of hair are curled with a curling iron, then allowed to cool down, and kept in place with hair spray.* **3** *Romantic: Roll the hair on medium-size curlers; when dry, shape with fingers only.* **4** *Wild and straggly: Apply styling wax to the blow-dried hair; part the hair in zigzag fashion. If necessary, straighten the hair with a curling iron.* **5** *Businesslike: Roll the hair back on medium-size curlers. Comb back, using styling gel.* **6** *Evening: Fasten the curls at the back of head with pins into a clump. Straighten the front part with gel and pull it across to the side, beginning at the side part.*

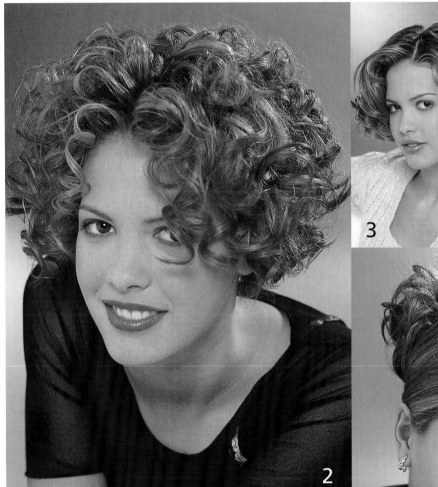

2

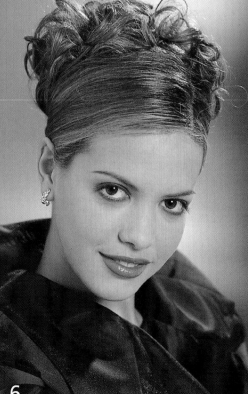

3

4

6

The cut:
A chin-length bob whose sides are all of one length. The top layer is shorter towards the back and is gently layered so it will turn under

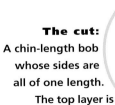

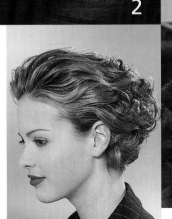

5

7 *Rounded look: Strengthen hair with volumizing mousse; create tension by blow-drying over a round brush.* **8** *Smart: Part hair zigzag-fashion and blow- dry hair to make it straight.* **9** *Nostalgic: Comb damp hair close to the head with styling gel. Using a comb and the side of the hand, shape into waves. Turn ends into a 6-shaped curl. Hold with hair spray.* **10** *Turned up: Blow-dry ends over a small round brush towards the outside; hold with hair spray.* **11** *1960s look: Part hair on side, above forehead; smooth out with gel wax. Roll hair in the back up in curlers; when dry, tease.* **12** *Hot:*

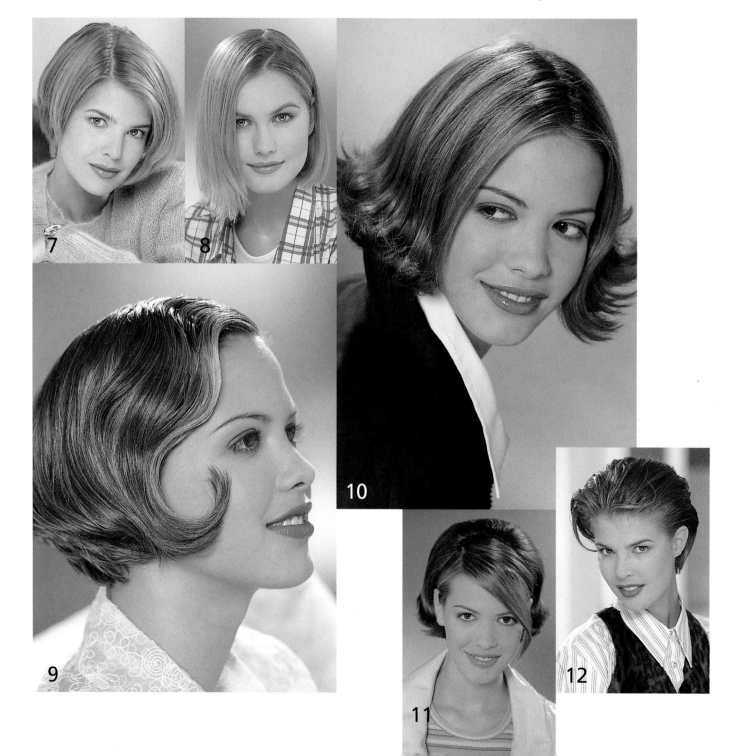

Apply styling gel and style, using all ten fingers, pulling hair back. A few strands from the top layer are pulled forward.
13 Extravagant: Part hair on the side, comb straight back behind the ears. Pull two strands from the top layer forward and hold with gel. **14** Full: Roll hair on large curlers, brush out opposite to the direction of growth, tease lightly.
15 Girlish look: A short middle part; tease at the back. Put gel on the sides and comb close to the head, behind the ears. **16** Curled: Comb hair up tightly and tie in two ponytails. With a curling iron, make small curls.
17 Waves: Add volume to this pageboy by rolling hair on large rollers. Massage styling gel into ends.
18 Boyish style: Blow-dry hair back. With a styling brush and volumizing mousse, create height in front by pulling the hair up above the scalp.

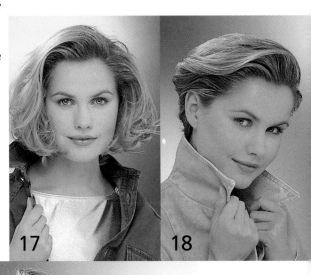

17

18

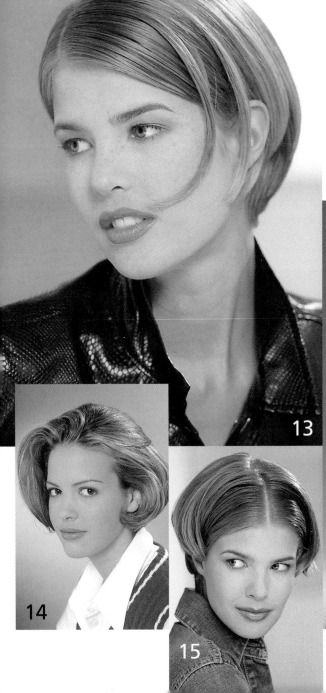

13

14

15

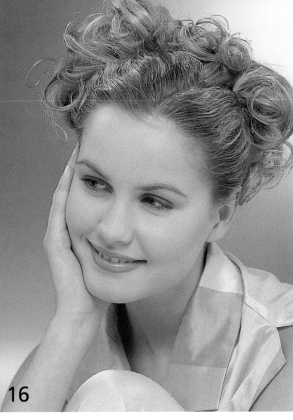

16

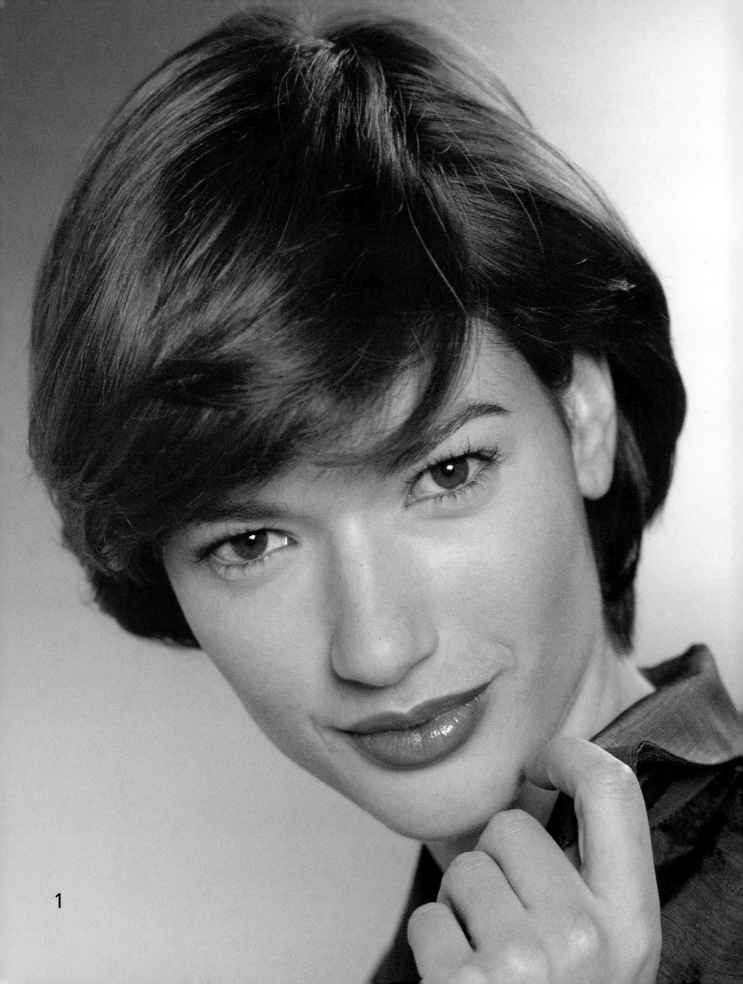

1

MEDIUM

The cut:
Short with a long
top layer. Bangs, neck, and
sides are carefully layered.
Overall fullness

3 *1950s look:
Part hair on
the left and the
right; pull the
bangs to the side.
Hold the hair in place
with hair spray.* **4** *Daring:
Blow-dry forward, tousle
ends with gel.* **5** *Cool: Add*

*gel, comb all hair back,
and blow-dry the neck
ends out and up.* **6** *Ladylike: Part the hair on the
side. Shape it at the
forehead with a curling
iron into a tuft. Apply gel
to the sides and comb
them close to the head.*

7 *Soft look: Part the hair
at the side, use large
curlers, and then blow-
dry.* **8** *Curls: Roll the hair
on heated curlers; when
cool, use the fingers to
tousle individual locks.
Secure the style with
styling gel.*

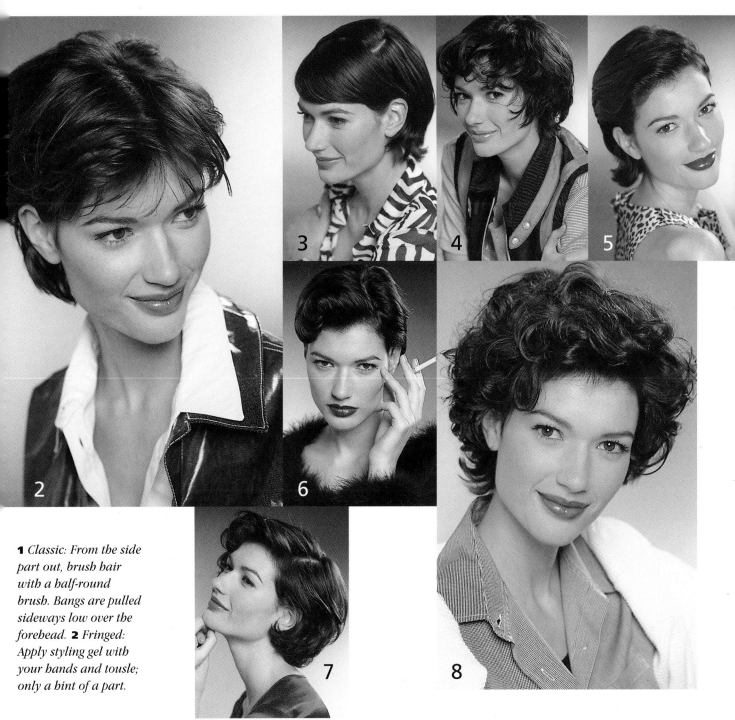

1 *Classic: From the side
part out, brush hair
with a half-round
brush. Bangs are pulled
sideways low over the
forehead.* **2** *Fringed:
Apply styling gel with
your hands and tousle;
only a hint of a part.*

The cut: Shoulder-length hair with blunt cut. In front it's slightly shorter

1 *Turning under: Blow-dry hair down over a round brush in separate layers.*
2 *Mini knots: Twist thin individual locks at the top of your head on themselves and secure with pins.*

3 *Romantic: Curl hair with curling papers. In back, roll hair into a small french roll.* **4** *Spiral curls: Apply styling gel and curl individual locks with a curling iron.*

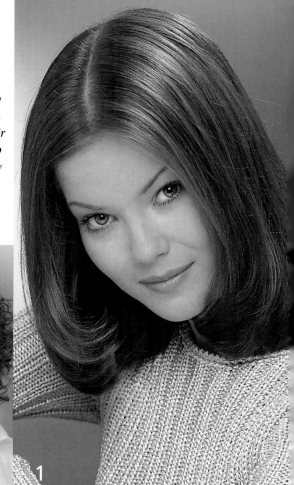

2

3

4

1

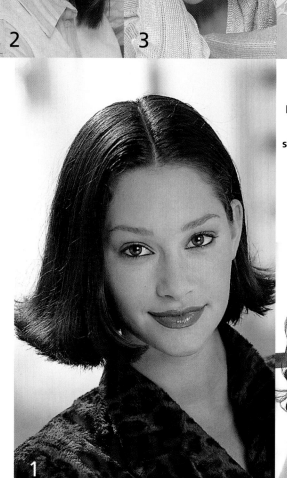

The cut: Hair is slightly longer than chin length and becomes progressively shorter towards the back. Hair ends will turn up almost by themselves

1 *Classic: Blow-dry, turning ends outwards around a round brush.*
2 *Playful: Roll hair on medium-thick curlers and tie them at the neck.*

3 *Fluffy curls: Apply styling liquid, use curling papers, and let dry overnight.* **4** *Piled high: Top layer is slightly teased and then casually pinned on top of the head.*

1

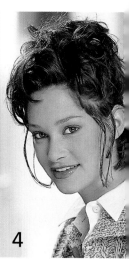

2

3

4

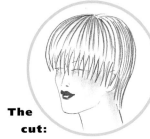

The cut:
Shaped evenly, a bit shorter in the front. Long top layer with full bangs, ends slightly layered

1 *Mushroom cut: Blow-dry the hair over a round brush, starting at the crown.*
2 *Punk style: Divide the hair into individual locks, twist them at the base, and clip them in place.*

Tease the ends and comb back; hold them in place with hair spray. **3** *Perfection: Blow-dry the hair to create body. Make a high part, add styling gel, and turn the locks*

towards face.
4 *Glamorous look: Apply gel and push the hair into waves in sections with the edge of your hand; secure them with long clips. Comb out the hair carefully.*

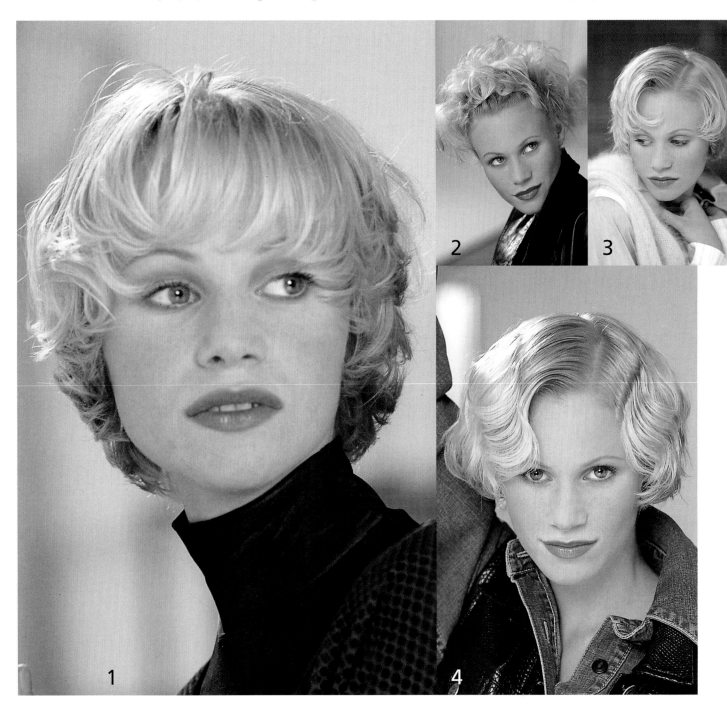

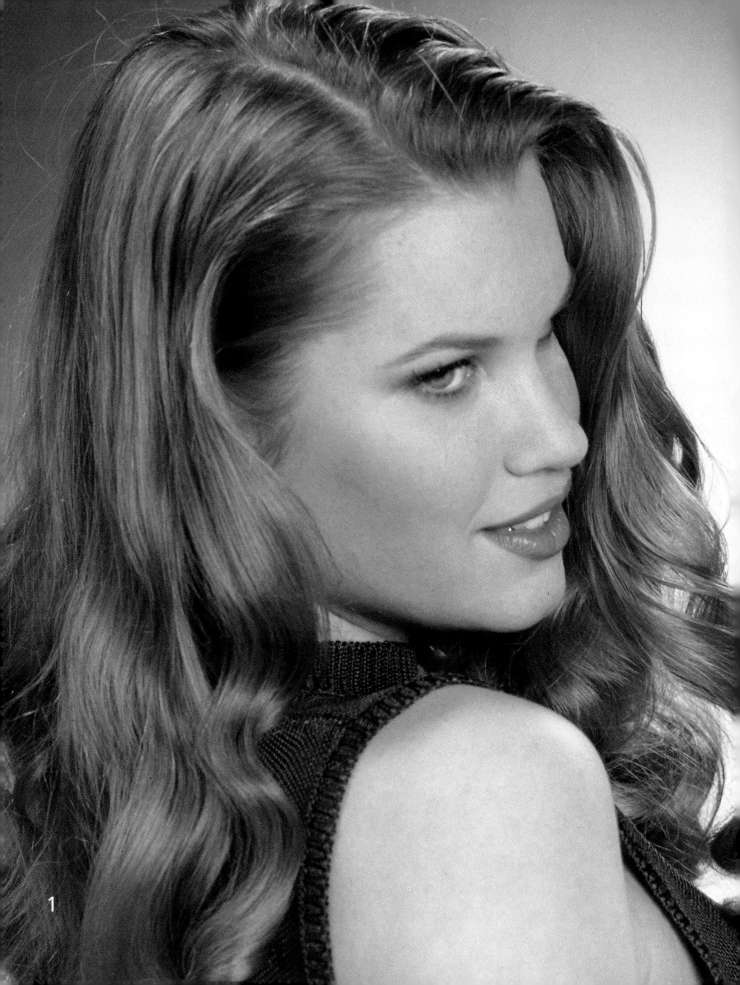

LONG *styles*

1 *Soft waves: Roll hair on heated curlers up to temple height.* **2** *Casually pinned up: Hair above forehead is pushed up. Sides are turned and pinned on top of head in indi-* *vidual locks. Hair in the back is casually turned under into a french roll.* **3** *Gracefully looped: Hair is pulled up, tied together at the crown, and divided into two parts,* *which are loosely arranged, crossing over in front.* **4** *Corkscrew curls: Hair is rolled up on heated curlers and not combed out. Each curl is pinned and sprayed with hair* *spray.* **5** *Beautifully simple: Part hair in the middle, apply styling lotion, comb back close to the head and tie behind the ears. Wind one lock around the tie to hide it.*

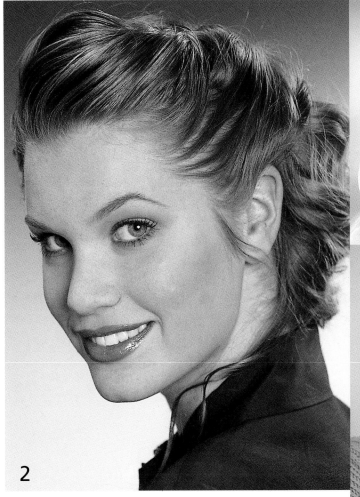

3

4

2

The cut:
An even blunt cut to
below shoulder length.
Only the ends in front are
slightly layered

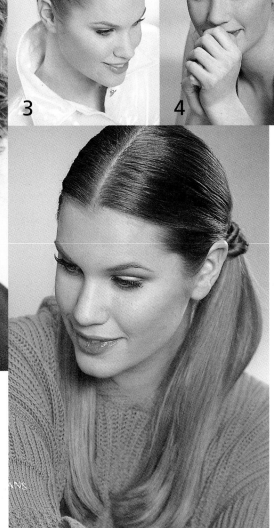

5

6 *Party look: Comb the hair close to the head with styling gel; gather at the neck with combs. Curl the ends around your finger and pin in place.*

7 *Teenage style: Blow-dry hair; push back with a flexible zigzag comb.*

8 *Hot: Divide hair into* individual locks at the crown, tie into loose knots, and pin in place. Tease the ends.

9 *Fashionably smooth: Part the hair relatively* low on the side and comb low over the forehead; secure behind the ear. Hold in place with hair spray.

10 *Movie-star waves:* Roll the hair on medium-size rollers up to ear height. When it is dry, style the ends over a round brush.

11 *Beautifully simple:*

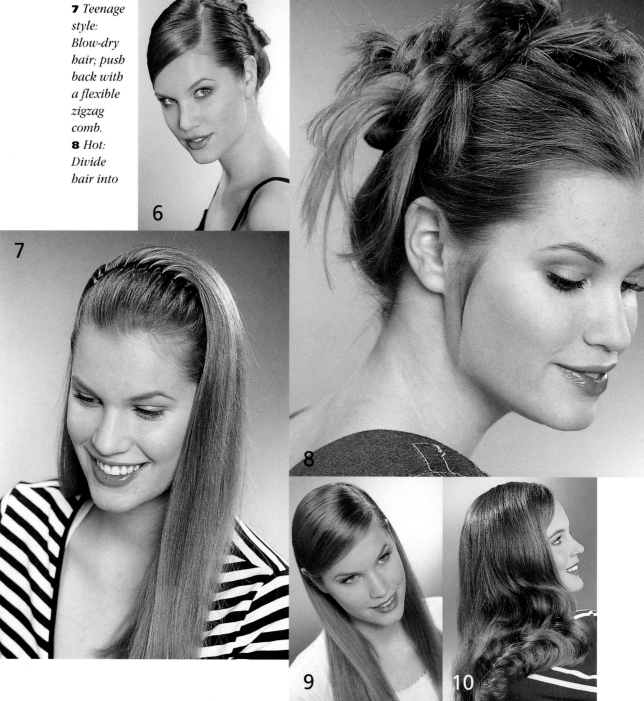

Part the hair high on the side, moisten with styling lotion, and blow-dry it flat. **12** Distinct profile: Pull the hair back loosely, fold the middle under casually, and pin in place. **13** Mini snails: Part the hair in zigzag fashion. Tie the left and right parts into ponytails. Divide each ponytail into three sections, tightly twist each section, and pin all three sections together in place above the ear. **14** Ponytail: Tie the hair in a ponytail at the crown and wrap a small scarf around it at the base for decoration.

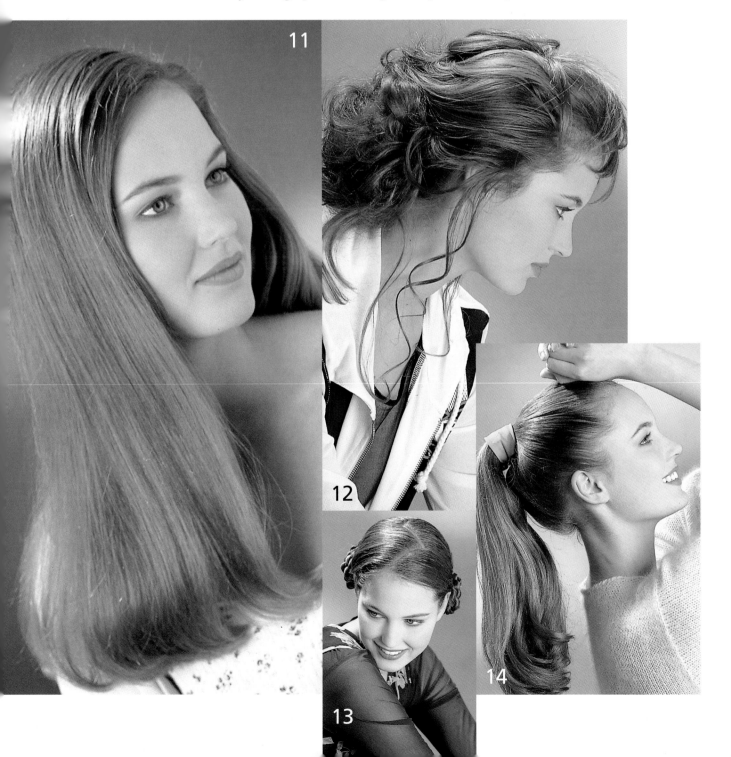

The cut:
Hair is blunt-cut to below shoulder length all around, except in front, where it is freely layered. The cut should follow the natural wave

1 *Front wave: Bend head down; blow-dry hair. Dampen hair in front with styling gel and, with a vent brush, pull up while blow-drying.*

2 *Striking: Pull hair back taut at the base of neck, pull once through an elastic and a second time pull only halfway through to create a loop.* **3** *Middle part: For more volume, blow-dry one lock at a time, turning each* around a brush up to ear height. **4** *Refined: Part hair, starting at one ear and going straight across to the other ear. Fold the back into a french roll and pull out a few strands. Divide the hair in front in half and twist into loose loops.*

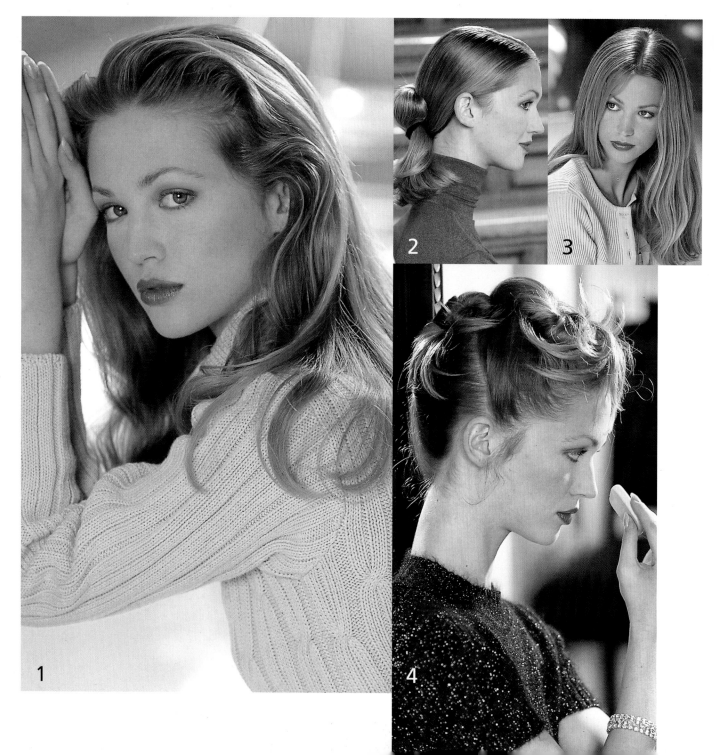

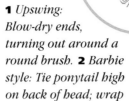

The cut: Angled contour from chin down to shoulder length. Ends are feathered

1 *Upswing: Blow-dry ends, turning out around a round brush.* **2** *Barbie style: Tie ponytail high on back of head; wrap at the base with a thick lock of hair.* **3** *Piled high: Divide ponytail in two sections, twist each lock separately, and pile one on top of the another; pin in place.* **4** *Turned under: Curl ends in and forward with a curling iron in front.*

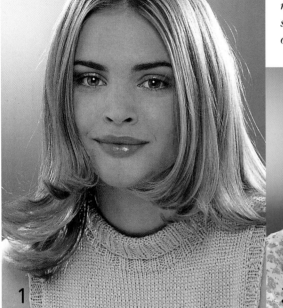

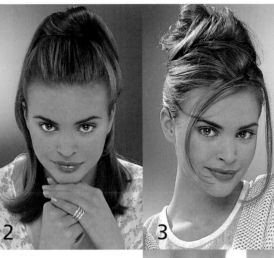

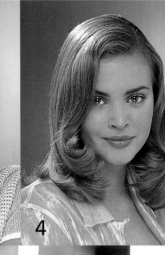

The cut: Below shoulder length; a somewhat rounded contour; gently layered ends

1 *Twisted ends: Roll hair in curlers; when dry, shape front over a round brush, holding brush vertically.* **2** *Romantic: Smooth and close to head in front; in back, braided once and then tied together.* **3** *Super mane: Roll small individual locks in curlers; then massage styling gel into hair.* **4** *Festive: High ponytail; wrap the elastic with a lock of hair.*

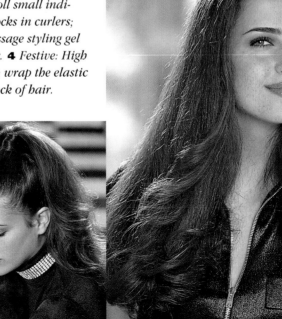

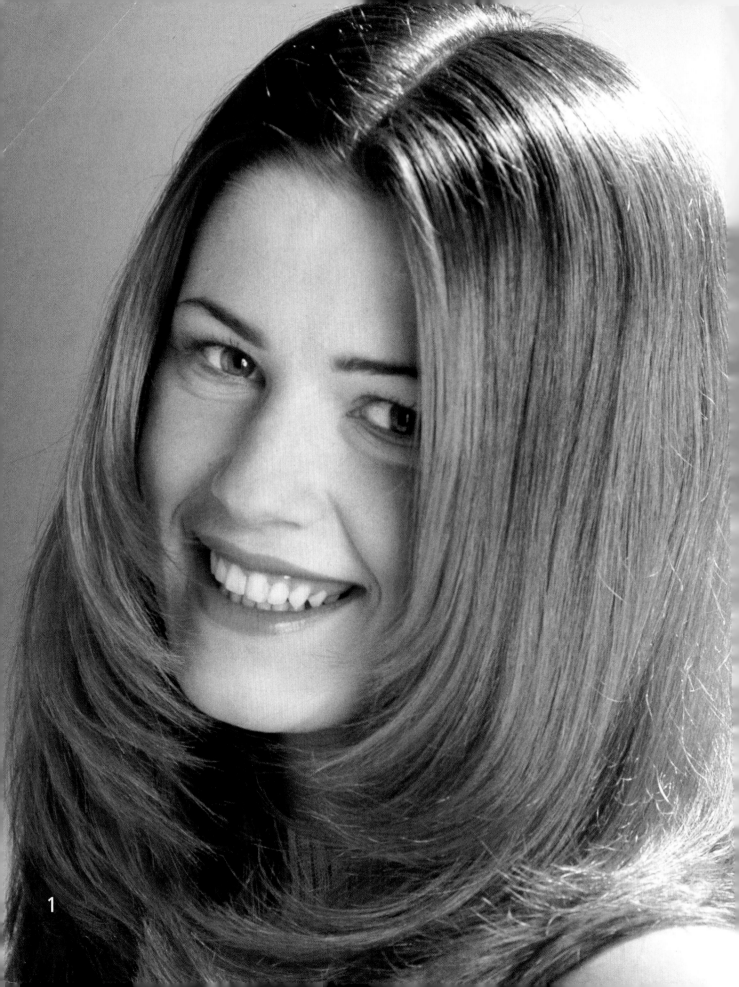

The cut: Below shoulder length straight hair with a clearly layered contour starting at the height of the mouth. Ideal for thick hair

curlers; when dry, the large curls are draped in front of the knot. **3** Turned under: First roll the hair on thick curlers; when it is dry, turn the ends

under, using the hair dryer. **4** Mane with fringes: Part the hair irregularly and tease heavily on the top and in back. **5** Western girl: Tie pigtails on the sides, allowing some strands to fall across the face.

6 Glamour look: Roll hair on thick curlers and brush out over the head with the head bent down. Shake into place. **7** Piled up: Randomly pile hair up on the top of the head; then pin in place.

1 Middle part: Blow-dry the hair flat over a round brush, turning the ends inside.
2 Loose curls: The hair in the back is pulled up and shaped into a knot. The front is rolled on thick

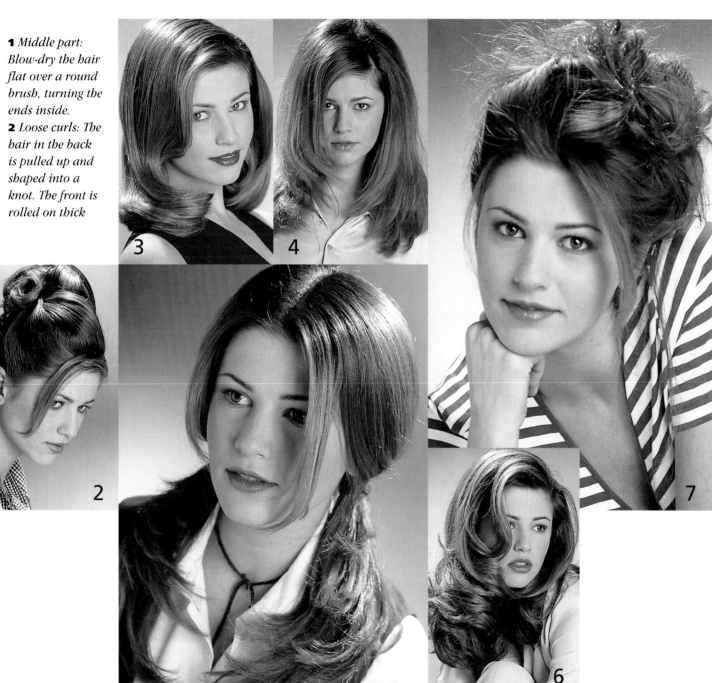

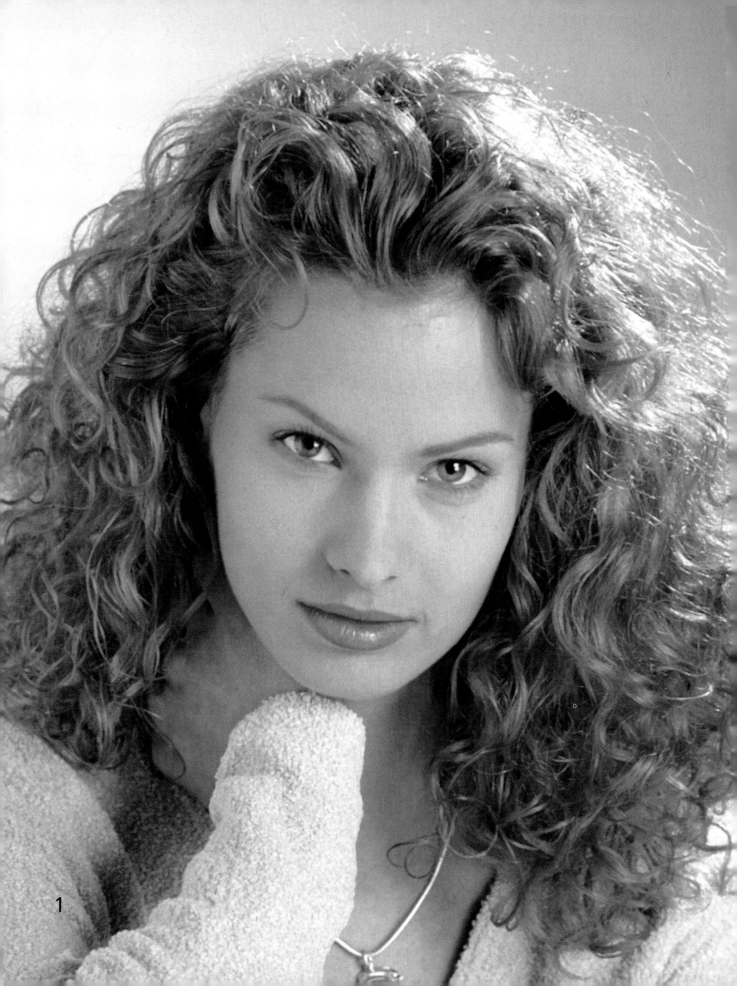

1

LONG CURLY *styles*

1 *Mop of curls: Blow-dry with diffuser, scrunching hair as it dries.* **2** *Soft mane: Roll hair on thick curlers. When dry, add* styling gel and shape into curls with fingers. **3** *Squash waves: Apply gel to the front part of hair and push into waves; use hair spray* to keep shape. Back part: Fold into french roll and pin. **4** *Piled high: twist locks of hair above forehead into curls; fasten with pins.* The rest is held in place with small combs. **5** *Narrow: Hair on each side is pulled back and pinned at the back of the head.*

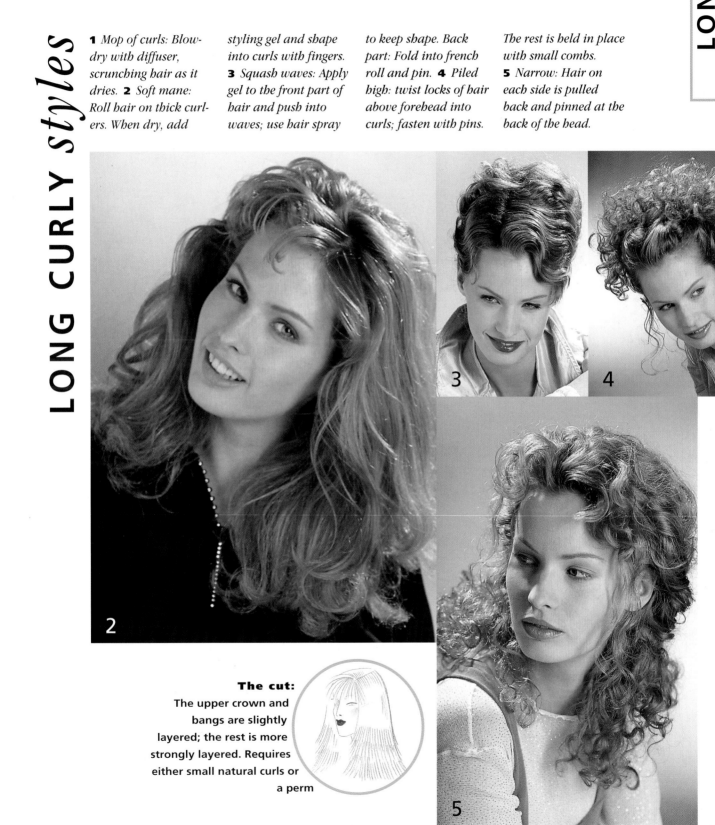

The cut: The upper crown and bangs are slightly layered; the rest is more strongly layered. Requires either small natural curls or a perm

6 *Corkscrew curls: Individual locks are curled into corkscrew curls with a curling iron. Bangs are pulled across flat, close to head, and pinned.*
7 *1970s style: Blow-dry hair, keeping it straight; separate hair at crown from hair in back and tie in ponytail. Wind a braided lock of hair around it.*
8 *Smooth: Dampen hair with styling liquid; blow-dry, pulling*
to keep hair straight.
9 *Piled high: Tie curls together on top of head and pull them apart with your fingers.*
10 *Glamorous: With*
gel, a comb, and back of hand, shape waves in front. Hold with long clips to dry. Curls are fluffed out with a diffuser.

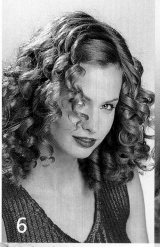

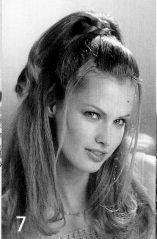

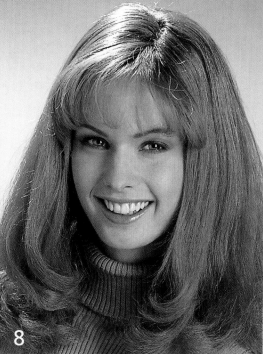

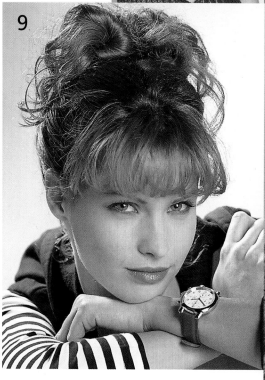

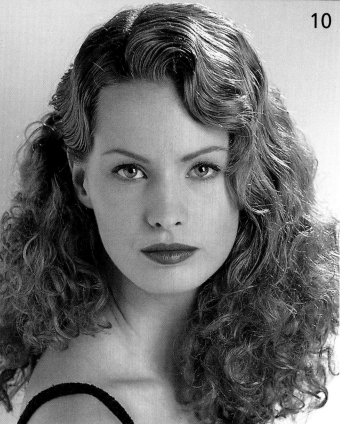

The cut:
An even blunt cut all around, below shoulder length hair—for natural curls that are not too thick

1 *Crushed curls: Slightly dry hair with head bent over; use a diffuser. Add styling gel and massage well into curls.* **2** *Curly head: Twist hair at top of head into small snail shapes; pin in place. Curly ends are randomly pulled out, kept loose.* **3** *Hollywood: Roll hair on thick curlers; when dry, comb out gently. Ends are styled all around with a round brush (see pages 84–85).*

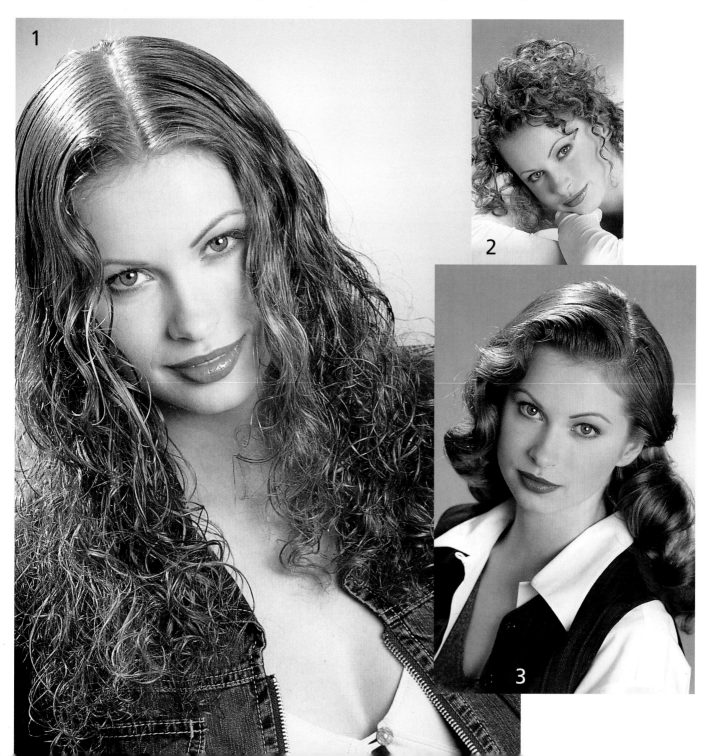

WHAT HAIR LIKES...

Three things are important to have your hairstyle stay and be carefree: a haircut that fits your type of hair, which is reshaped on a regular basis; proper care for your kind of hair, and as little mechanical and chemical stress as possible.

Good: A Super Cut

If hair is cut properly, a hairstyle will stay without needing much help from a brush, a hair dryer, or curlers. This not only saves time; it is also much healthier for the hair, because it is spared loss of moisture and won't have to suffer the consequences of mechanical manipulation. This is particularly important when hair is shampooed daily. Which haircut is the proper one can only be determined by the hairstylist. He or she will assess carefully how your hair falls naturally, whether it has cowlicks, how thin or thick it is, whether the surface of each hair is rough or smooth, if the ends are intact and not split. In any case, it is advisable to carefully listen to the recommendations of a professional person, even if the person does not tell you what you hoped to hear. If your hair isn't the right kind for your "dream hairstyle," daily care quickly can turn into a nightmare.

Regular reshaping also is important. Because each hair grows at a different rate, even the best haircut will be less than perfect after four weeks.

Good: Things That Make Your Hair Smooth

This could be an acid rinse used after shampooing, rinsed out immediately, or a spray lotion that remains in the hair. (Or a moisturizing lotion when your hair feels rough to the touch, or volumizing lotion if your hair is fine and needs more body and sheen.) These lotions can be used as a preventative each time you shampoo your hair without overdoing it. They add a fine film to the surface, making the hair soft, and protect hair from the heat of the hair dryer and other styling methods. These protective effects can be increased with regular treatments using more intensive products. The latter are usually left on for ten minutes and contain substances that not only smooth the hair surface, but penetrate to strengthen the hair. How often should these products be used? Depending on the state of your hair, do this every 2 to 3 weeks.

Good: Drying Hair the Gentle Way

Tip 1: First, without using a brush, bend over and go through your hair with your fingers, as a kind of predrying method. The hair dryer should be set at its highest level. When the hair is only slightly damp, reduce heat to the lowest level.

Tip 2: Don't hold the hair dryer too close to the hair, and always let the air move from the roots out towards the ends. But the best thing is to let your hair air-dry naturally as frequently as possible.

Good: High-Quality Tools

Combs, brushes, and curlers that are in bad shape can damage the surface of each individual hair. Daily exposure to less-than-perfect tools will make styling difficult, resulting in loss of sheen and unruliness. First principle of brushing: the ends of the bristles should not look as if they have been broken off; they must be smooth and rounded. A combination of natural and manmade bristles is best. Round brushes work best when long and short bristles are combined; hair can be brushed smoothly, keeping hairs from getting caught when you remove the brush. Check comb teeth for raised seams and rough spots. Only combs with smooth teeth are gentle to the hair. Do not use metal combs; good plastic is alright. If your hair is delicate, do not use curlers with brushes inside or self-stick rollers: only use velvet-covered rollers.

AND DOESN'T LIKE

Bad: Rough Combing

Hair is more vulnerable when it is wet, because water expands the keratin inside each hair shaft, and rough handling in that state weakens its structure. Pulling a comb through your hair after shampooing can easily overstretch it. That—in combination with other "sins"—will turn hair into straw and make it coarse. A comb with extra wide-set teeth is particularly important for long hair. Hold wet hair halfway down and start combing or brushing from there on down; do not start combing at the roots, but rather at the ends. Carefully untangle from below, moving slowly up.

Bad: Drastic Color Changes

This refers particularly to changing from dark to light. While extreme lightening of hair is not a problem with today's modern products when it is done by an experienced professional, the hair will still lose a lot of pigment, which means much of its substance, until the new, lighter color develops. Only very healthy, thick hair will survive such a procedure with a minimum of damage. And since dark hair needs frequent touch-ups, even under favorable circumstances, prob-lems are bound to arise. In any case, drastic changes should never be done at home.

Bad: When Hair Is Overtreated

That, too, happens: hair also suffers from too much care and reaches a state where styling becomes difficult and natural bounce is lost. This happens because rinses and treatments, used too often, create a build-up, depositing certain substances on the surface of the hair. How much hair care is suffi-cient without creating buildup differs from one person to the next. Experiment and you will find the right balance for you. **Rule of thumb:** One treatment a week, and rinsing or using a conditioner after each, or every other shampooing, depending on the state of your hair. In case of build-up, use a neutral shampoo that has no additional substances for awhile.

Bad: Perming and Coloring at the Same Time

Besides the fact that doing both of these on the same day would take a long time, every professional would discourage the customer from coloring and perming together. Hair needs a couple of weeks to recover from the effects of a perm; coloring or tinting will not turn out as well if you do them together, because the hair structure has been loosened. And the opposite is also true: if you have freshly colored hair, it will negatively influence the results if you perm immediately afterwards. For that reason, allow at least two weeks between treatments. You risk injuring your hair otherwise.

Bad: When Hair Has Been Exposed to Too Much Sun

Particularly when hair is wet, the sun's rays act like peroxide, bleaching the hair. In case of light hair that is strong and healthy, exposure to sun can create a charming effect, but when the hair is sensitive, fine, or already has been stressed (e.g., hair that has been colored or permed), the effect is usually fatal. The hair loses its smooth-ness, the colors lose their original tone, a perm turns hair into straw. A good solution is to cover your hair as a matter of course with a hat or a scarf when you are in the sun. If that is not possible, a presun lotion sprayed on the hair before exposure is protection against loss of elasticity as well as against ultraviolet rays. In the evening, shampoo hair with an after-sun shampoo.

CHAPTER II

Volume: HOW TO

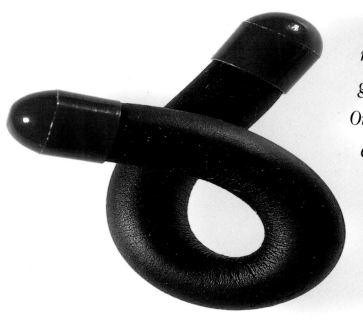

Do you need a hairstyle that
makes more out of thin hair or
gives your hair a bigger profile?
On the next twelve pages, you can
choose whichever one you like.
Immediately following that
are hairstyles that can
be done in split seconds—
particularly good for
hair that gets greasy very
quickly or split ends that you
would like to hide.

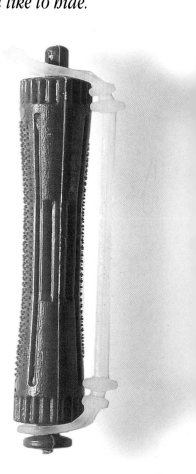

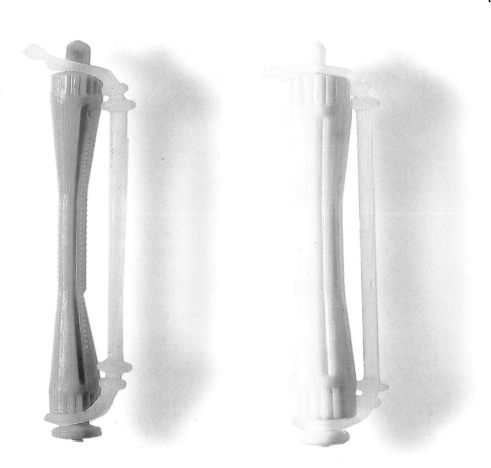

GIVE YOUR HAIR BODY

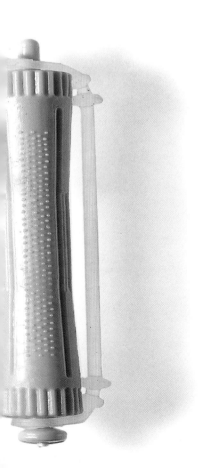
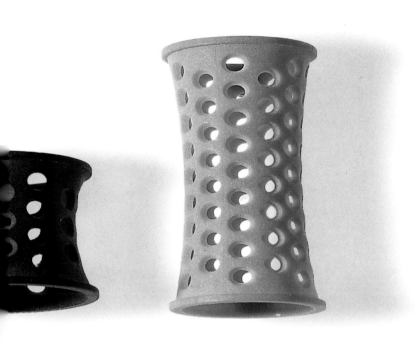
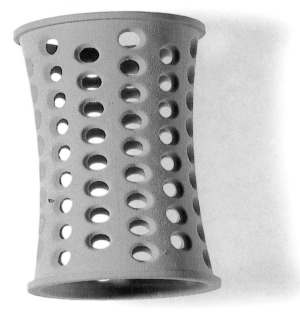
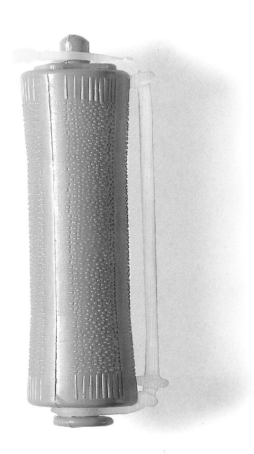
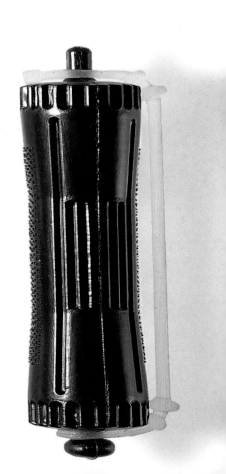

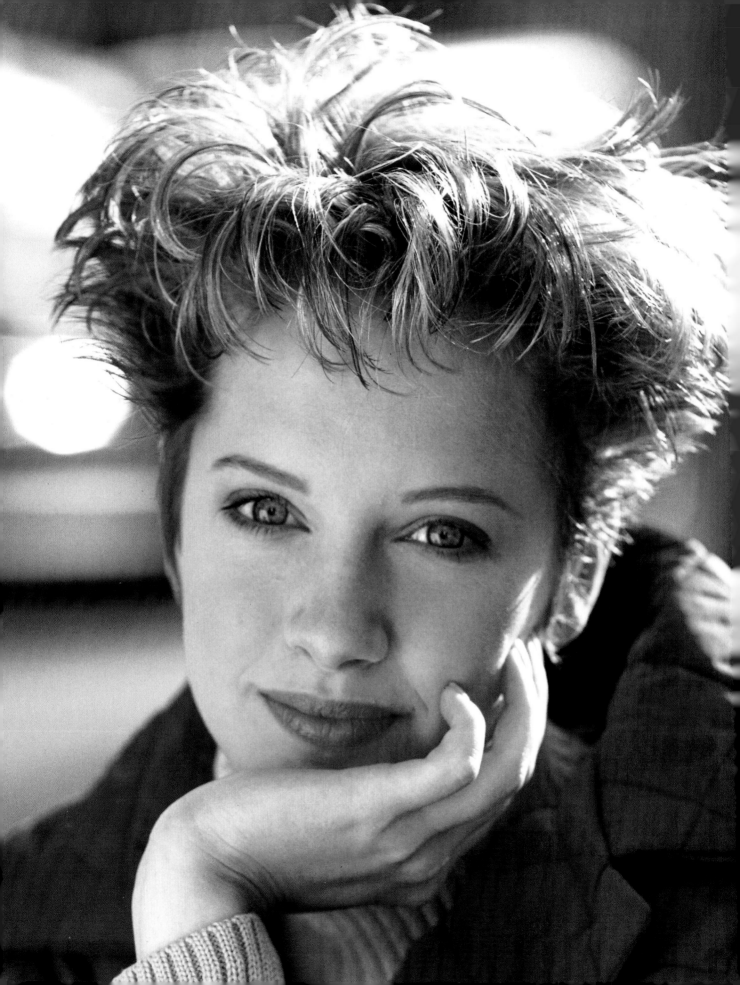

FULL SHORT *styles*

For full short hairstyles, the most important thing is to lift the hair off the scalp at the roots. To make the style last: use a volumizing mousse.

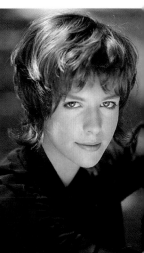

Well-layered ends give this bob good volume. One lock at a time, blow-dry hair over a vent brush, moving hair forward and up.

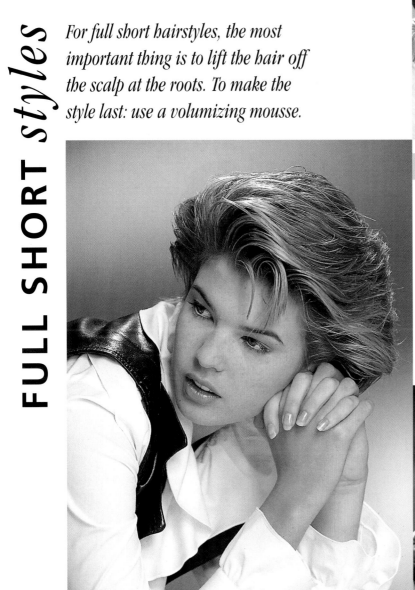

Short cut, layered towards the back. Blow-dry one lock at a time, moving back. Pull hair against growth direction at roots. Hold with hair spray.

The shorter the cut, the more volume. Blow-dry in layers around a large round brush. Pin top layer out of the way to blow-dry layers beneath.

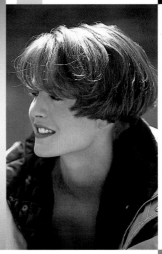

This cut creates casual fullness by featherlike shaping of contours. Hair is close to head on sides and in back, making the crown look fuller. This style is good for thin, fine hair.

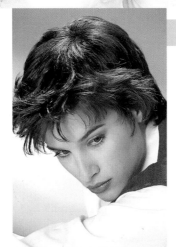

Photo at left: *To be sure hair stays above the scalp at the roots, especially in front, bend head down and pull hair away from the head with fingers as you blow-dry, section by section. Finger-shape ends with styling gel or mousse.*

Here the upturned ends give the impression of volume. Massage mousse into hair and blow-dry upwards around a medium-size round brush. Hold with spray.

The easiest solution for adding volume to short hair: a perm with small curls. Let dry naturally for zero work. Massage volumizing mousse into hair.

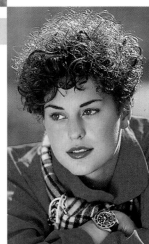

A bob permed with large curlers. After shampooing, add volumizing mousse and shape with all ten fingers. Let air-dry naturally, moving your fingers through the hair as it dries; shake head often.

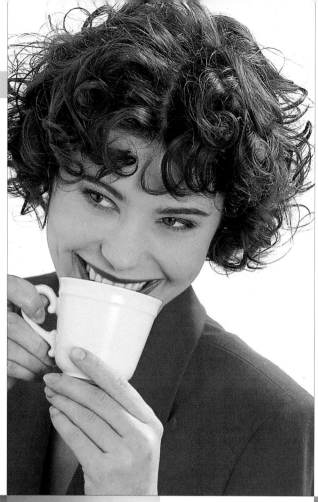

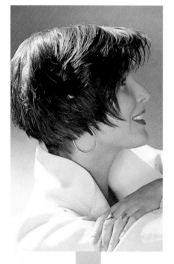

A layered, short cut emphasizing fringes all around. Volume at the back is created by blow-drying in layers over a round brush from underneath up.

Photo at right: *Here the remnants of a perm provide casual fullness overall. Blow-dry hair with head bent down. Add volume to the fringe-cut contour with volumizing mousse and blow-drying (it is best to use a diffuser); use fingers to pull hair away from head.*

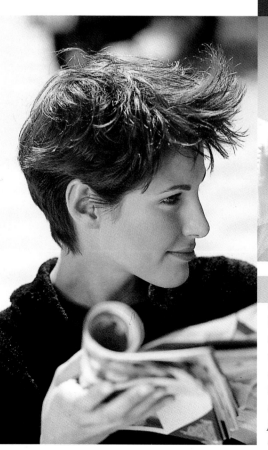

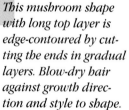

This mushroom shape with long top layer is edge-contoured by cutting the ends in gradual layers. Blow-dry hair against growth direction and style to shape.

A classic cut for volume: A very low part; the top layer is kept long over very short sides.

The close-cropped neck creates a beautiful full silhouette, even without any styling aids. The fringelike bangs in the front are dried upwards, providing fullness and movement.

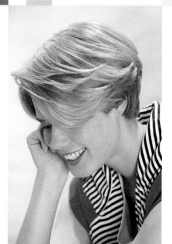

Hair is rolled in locks on heated curlers and allowed to cool. Comb out with a wide-tooth comb and shape carefully; hold with styling liquid or gel.

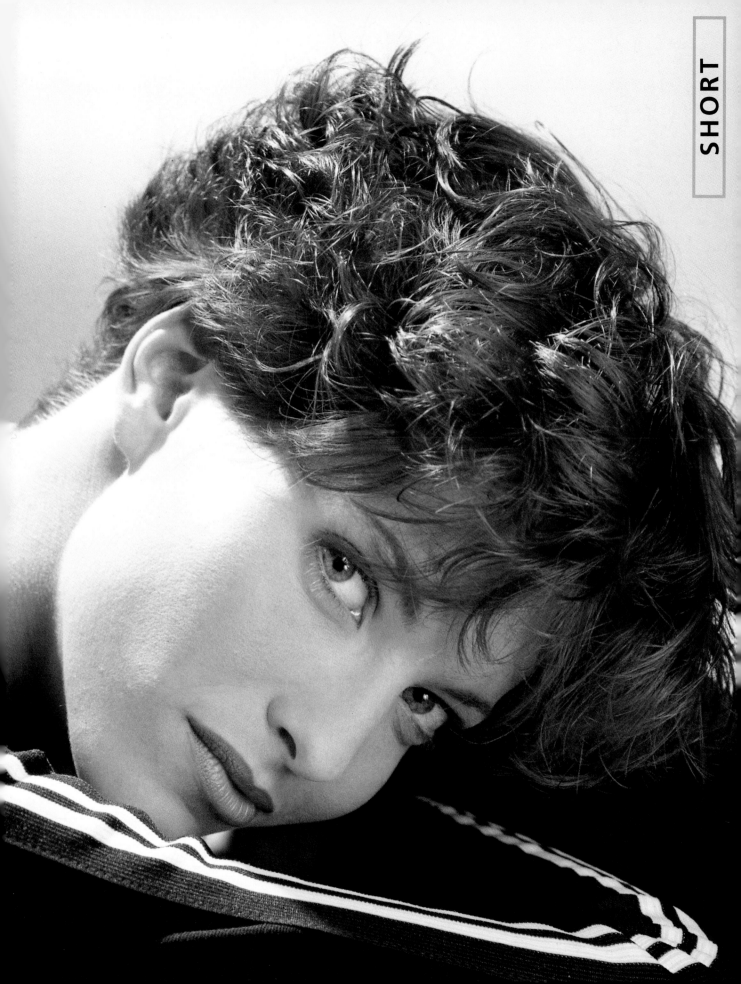

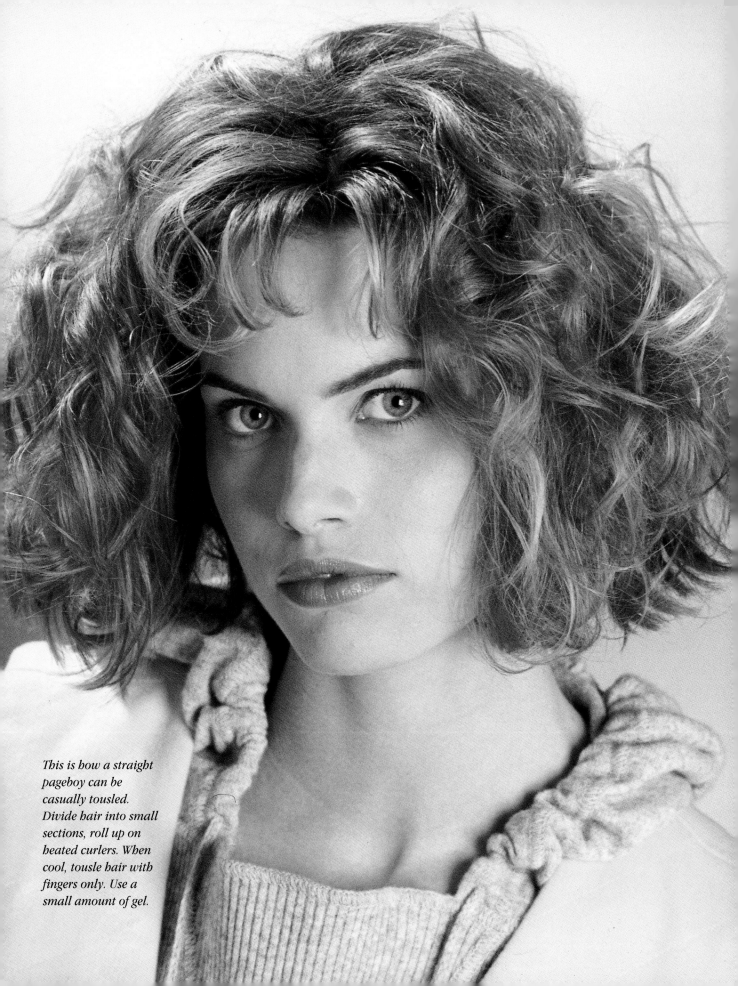

This is how a straight pageboy can be casually tousled. Divide hair into small sections, roll up on heated curlers. When cool, tousle hair with fingers only. Use a small amount of gel.

MEDIUM

FULL MEDIUM LENGTH *styles*

Most important tip for fullness with medium length hair: pin top layers out of the way and blow-dry hair in layers over a round or vent brush, working from the underneath layer up.

For this pageboy, contours are slightly layered, allowing the ends to support each other, so the volume created by blow-drying lasts.

For this shaggy look, the top layer is layered and the hair is rolled up on curlers.

Volume at the roots: Chin-length hair rolled on large heated rollers; cool down and brush out with a coarse brush with the head bent down.

Fullness—an illusion! The trick: hair parted in middle with long, angled bangs. For optimum tension and volume, roll each hair section over the brush, blow-dry, and leave on brush until cold.

To give a classic pageboy more fullness, slightly layer the top layer. Blow-dry, first with head bent forward; then dry in layers.

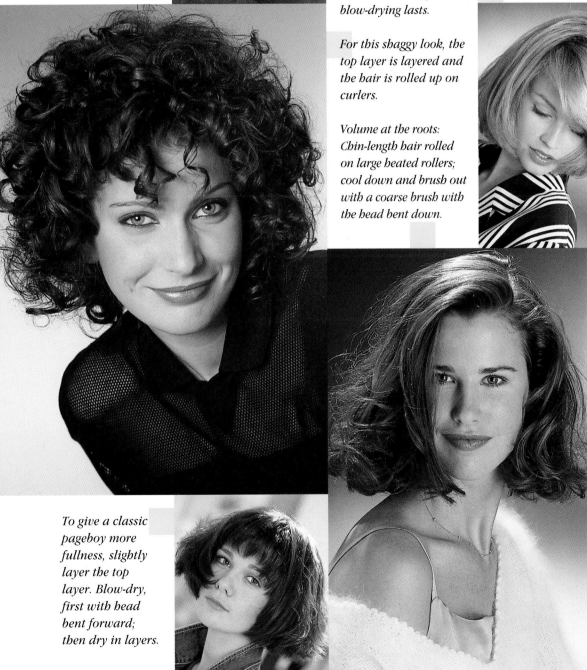

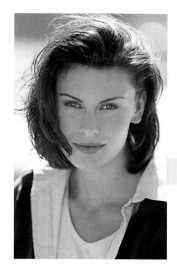

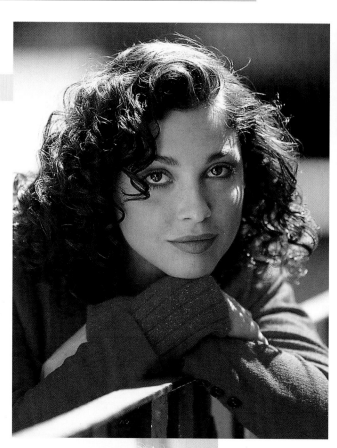

Tamed volume for natural curls: layered cut throughout the whole length. At roots combed close to the head. Apply styling gel or mousse. Blow-dry with a diffuser.

For this pageboy, the hair above the forehead has been slightly layered. That makes it easier for the hair to remain high, giving the impression of top fullness. The front is held with styling gel.

Style and fullness for natural waves: Top layer is one length throughout, hair at the back of neck is layered. Let dry naturally, lifting the hair away from the scalp with both hands and shaking head often.

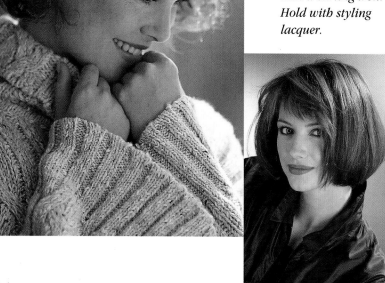

Curls galore for special occasions: Prepare hair by applying an extra strong hold styling product. Then curl hair, one lock at a time, from ends to the roots, vertically with a curling iron. Hold with styling lacquer.

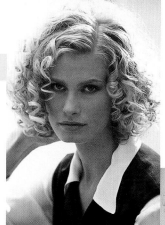

Natural or permed waves are cut in layers. Roll the hair on small curlers or rollers; and when it is com-pletely dry, tousle with fingers.

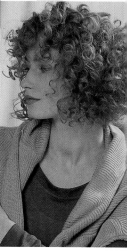

Volume trick for very straight hair. A side part is made high up, so a section of the hair that would have been flat hangs forward opposite the direction of growth.

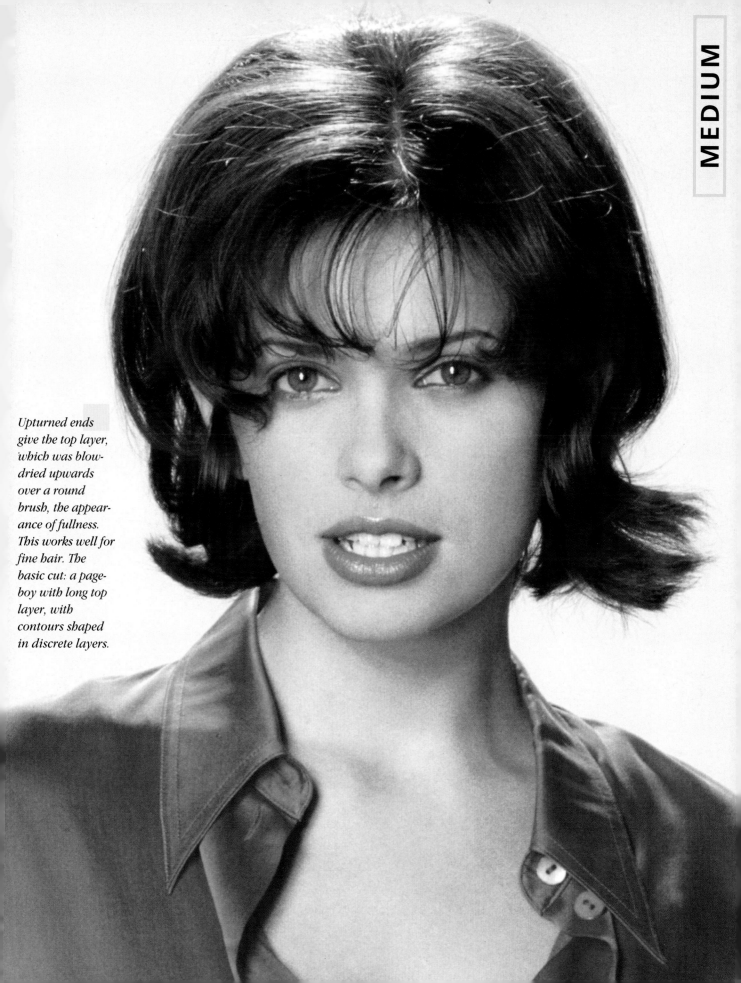

Upturned ends give the top layer, which was blow-dried upwards over a round brush, the appearance of fullness. This works well for fine hair. The basic cut: a page-boy with long top layer, with contours shaped in discrete layers.

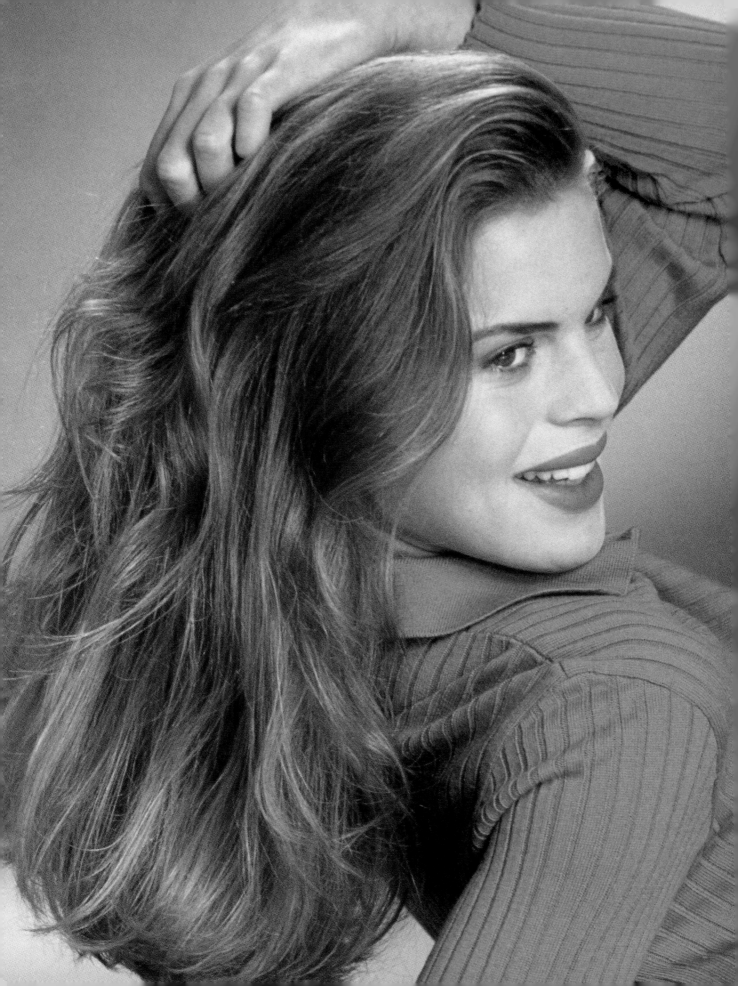

FULL LONG *styles*

Blunt-cutting ends and blow-drying hair with the head bent forward makes long hair immediately appear fuller. To have the hair at the roots stand up better, change your part often.

Volumizing mousse and extra large curlers are the secret of this full hairstyle. It works well with hair that is naturally slightly curly, or with permed hair.

A perm, with the top hair layered, is slightly teased in front, then pinned back.

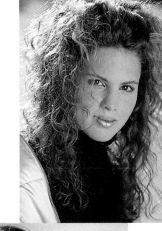

Layering hair in front takes off some weight. This makes it easier to lift hair in front and also makes turned-in, blow-dried ends more stable.

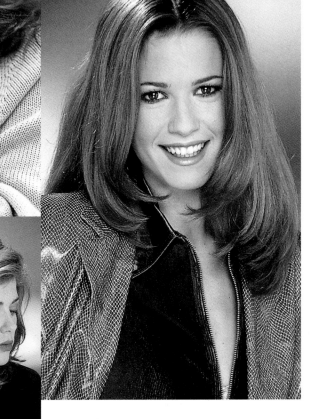

Photo at left: *Casual fullness is created by hair parted on the side, rolled on a few large rollers and, when completely dry, vigorously brushed out with the head bent down.*

The sides are layered, level with the tip of the nose, so that they turn in and fall forward almost by themselves. Add mousse and blow-dry with head bent down. Wind ends down over a round brush and blow-dry.

Here, bangs contribute to the impression of fullness. Add volumizing mousse to bangs and blow-dry the layered ends, turning down over a round brush.

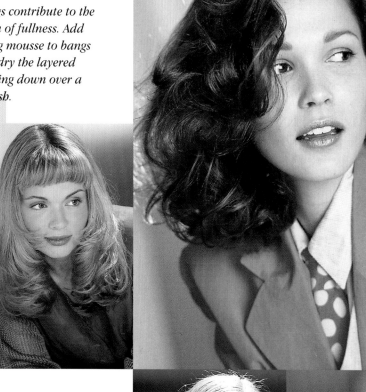

Full waves are formed by making low side part and combing the hair up over to the other side. The contour is slightly layered so it will look better.

Waves framing a face give the impression of fullness, even when there is little. Ends must be very well layered. Shape into curls with a curling iron. Add styling gel and pull curls down.

Movie-star waves always look lush. Roll hair on very thick curlers. Brush hair, turning the ends in (see pages 84–85).

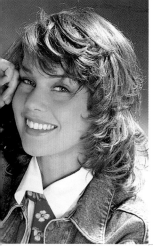

An age-old trick: Dampen the hair slightly and braid into many small braids. Allow to dry overnight. In the morning, undo the braids and ruffle with fingers.

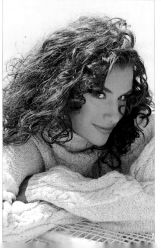

Casual body only in the lengths. Hair is rolled up to ear height on curlers or rolled on diagonally on folded paper napkins (knot the napkin ends). Dry hair gently, comb out with a wide-tooth comb.

Individual locks are blow-dried over a round brush and clipped into place. When completely dry, bend head down and tousle hair with fingers only.

STYLING FOR MORE BODY

It's possible to successfully lift the hair at the roots to add volume, even with fine, soft, or thin hair. Special styling techniques are the answer. Use products that give fullness and stability without adding weight.

Blow-drying hair against the direction of its growth creates volume for long and short hair, whether you let your hair dry naturally or use a hair dryer. Bend over, be sure to point the airflow away from the hair roots, and use a vent brush or fingers to move hair back and forth opposite to the direction of growth.

Tip 1: Lift hair straight up at roots when drying
One method is to spread your fingers; move them through hair, holding hair tightly, and pull hair away from the scalp; point the airflow away from roots. Then turn your hand up and over so that the hair is bent over the fingers. Continue blow-drying. (This works very well for the hair roots above the forehead.) For even better results, bend head forward and down. **Another method:** Use a vent brush instead of your fingers, and point the hair dryer away from the roots and opposite to the direction of growth.

Tip 2: Blow-dry your hair in stages
This trick works very well for medium-length hair, particularly for any type of pageboy. Clip the top layer out of the way and—starting at the neck and temples—blow-dry hair in sections over a round brush, pulling hair up, away from the scalp. This creates a stable foundation. Continue with the next layer, and proceed in the same way. Then blow-dry the top layer.

Always let hair cool down well. Why? Warm temperatures soften hair shafts. (If this weren't true, hair could not be shaped into curls or waves.) And the opposite is true: hair needs to cool down to keep its shape well. For that reason, do not remove the brush too soon when blow-drying. Keep the brush in place, turn the hair dryer away, and allow the hair to cool for a couple of seconds. This also applies for styling with a curling iron or heated curlers: the longer you let the hair cool down, the more stable the styling will be.

Tip 3: Use volume-building products
Shampoos, spray lotions, and intensive-care treatments that add volume surround the hair with a stabilizing film, making it stronger and increasing the distance between the individual hairs. Volumizing lotion is used after shampooing. It strengthens structurally weak hair with the amino acid cystine, very similar to the keratin present in hair; it also provides sheen. Volume-producing intensive treatments contain keratin peptide and silk protein, which provide fullness and stability without adding weight. Volumizing shampoo acts as a mild cleanser and leaves a fine film that strengthens hair, without adding weight.

Tip 4: Use setting lotion sparingly
More is not always better. Too much mousse and lotion—either for blow-drying hair or for styling—will be more likely to make

hair stiff than to curl it or give it volume. Use a dab of volumizing mousse the size of a walnut for short hair; use about double or triple that amount if you have longer hair.

Short hairstyles with the top layer distinctly layered, geometric cuts, and short bobs (pageboys) with blunt-cut contours are best for hair that needs additional body and volume (see pages 40–51). Medium-length hair should be cut just above the shoulders to avoid being too heavy. (The shorter the hair, the lighter it is, and the easier to add volume.) Very layered hair is not an advantage; hair loses volume when the ends are feathered and fall into each other.

Tip 5: How to apply hair spray
Simply spraying on hair spray—fogging it—won't help

much. That makes the top layer stiff, but doesn't stop a hairstyle from collapsing. With a short haircut, use hair spray only at the roots, before or after it is styled. If hair is longer, bend your head forward and shake it as you apply the hair spray. This creates flexible but stable volume. When hair is fine and needs more volume, a light styling spray works best.

Tip 6: Place curlers close together and roll hair up tightly
To give curly fullness to a casual pageboy and for long hair, use medium to large curlers. Here are some tips to make the volume you've added last:

1. Section hair into small locks and roll on curlers placed close together.
2. Roll hair tightly, pulling slightly against the direction of growth.
3. Before rolling a lock on a curler, spray on a small amount of setting lotion.
4. When brushing, add a dab of styling gel, or spray styling spray from below into the hair to give it more body.

Teasing hair immediately creates fullness. Divide the hair into locks and carefully tease hair with a

fine-tooth comb at the roots. Comb the top layer smooth with a wide-tooth comb. Fine, fragile hair should not be teased too much, because it roughens the surface of the hair shaft.

Tip 7: Casually pin up long hair
Fine, thin hair, worn long and straight, usually looks very sad. But when pinned up, it will appear to have more fullness, particularly if hair was rolled on curlers beforehand. Tease individual sections after the curlers have been removed, and hold with a small amount of hair spray. Then pin hair in place.

Tip 8: Get a permanent wave
Curly hair always seems to have more volume than straight hair, especially fine, thin hair. Volume can be created with a permanent wave if curls are allowed to dry naturally and the hair is tousled with all ten fingers, paying special attention to the scalp area, while hair is drying. Add a small amount of volumizing mousse and pull the ends outwards.

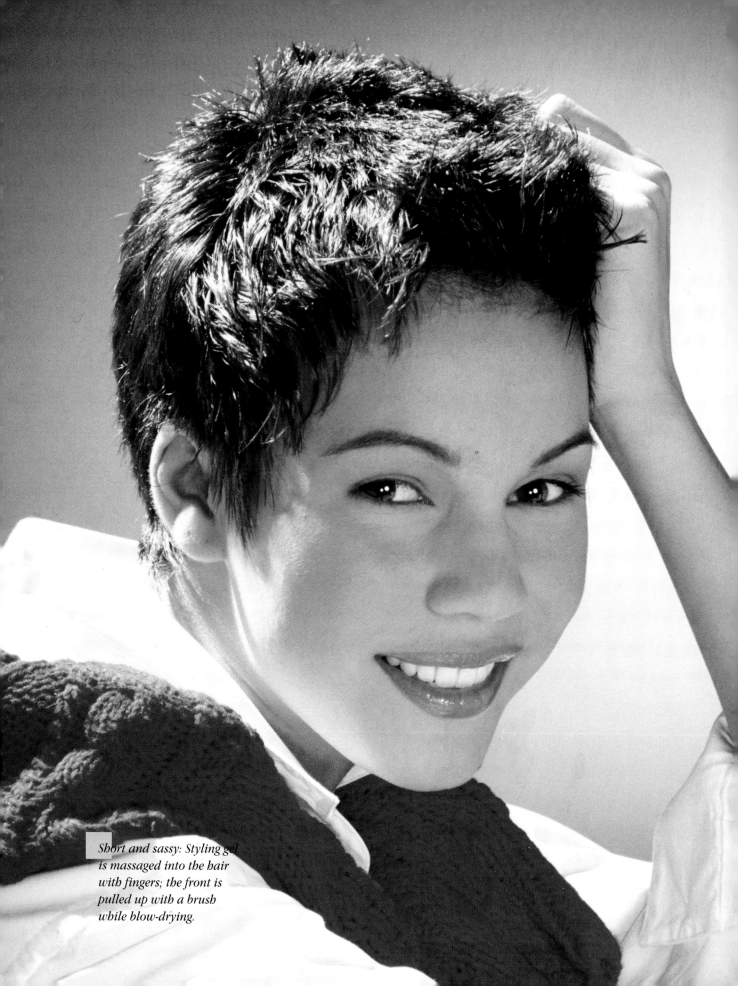

Short and sassy: Styling gel is massaged into the hair with fingers; the front is pulled up with a brush while blow-drying.

OIL-FIGHTING *quick styles*

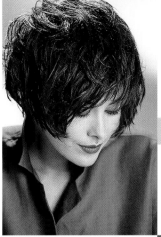

Layered cut: When blow-drying, move fingers through hair, pulling everything forward. Emphasize ends with styling gel.

Short, layered bob: Add styling liquid and blow-dry hair from the crown forward. Accentuate the top layer and ends with styling gel.

Bob with a perm: Let hair dry naturally; tousle hair now and then while it is drying. Work in a little styling gel to give shape to the curls.

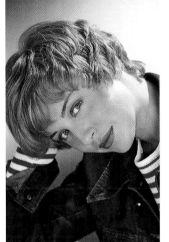

Garçon: Add styling gel to hair and comb it close to the head. Keep in place with two barrettes. Ends are pulled forward.

Zigzag part: Part hair in zigzag fashion and comb hair close to the head with the help of styling gel. Pull some strands in front of the ears.

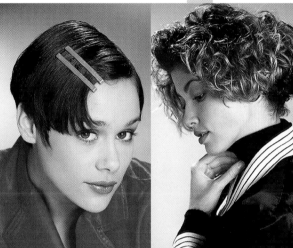

Here's a trick to prevent the greasy look: right after shampooing, add a small amount of gel to each lock. This will make a hairstyle last at least one day longer.

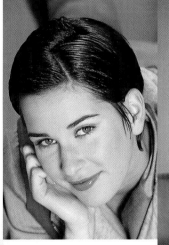

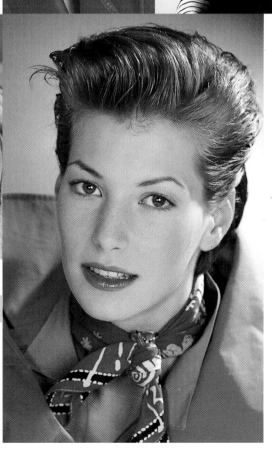

Rock 'n' roll: Add styling gel and comb hair back; push slightly forward. Hold with styling spray.

Shaggy: Add volumizing mousse and blow-dry back and forth. Ends are pulled away from the head and held in place with styling spray.

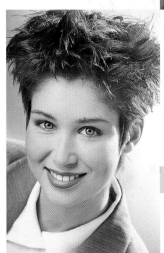

Pageboy with soft waves: Add styling liquid and blow-dry, pulling hair behind ears. Curl ends outward. Rub styling wax into the palms and gently smooth over.

Forehead waves: Add styling gel and comb. Pull hair up and forward in front, and keep in place with styling spray. Sides are tucked behind ears; hair in back is turned up.

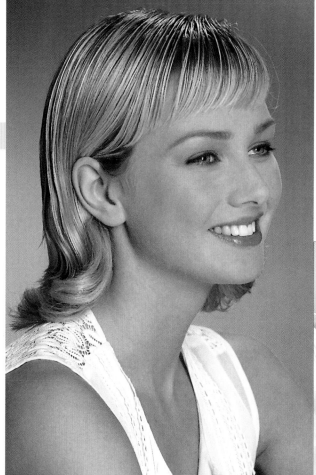

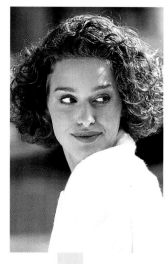

Curly pageboy: The unlayered hair is permed. Shampoo, add volumizing mousse, and let dry naturally.

Perm: top layer is slightly layered, so can move easily above the forehead. Let dry naturally; rub in styling gel.

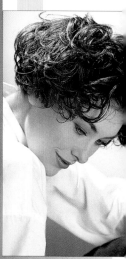

Gelled: A soft perm with a layered cut. Add a little styling gel while hair is still damp; tousle into shape.

Simply elegant: A bob without bangs, slightly teased over the forehead and combed behind the ears. Hold with a hint of styling spray or styling gel.

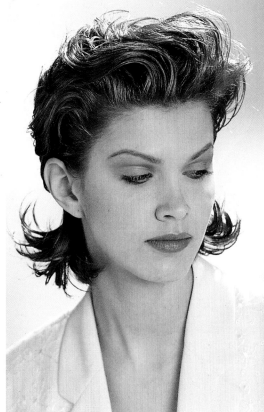

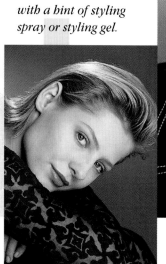

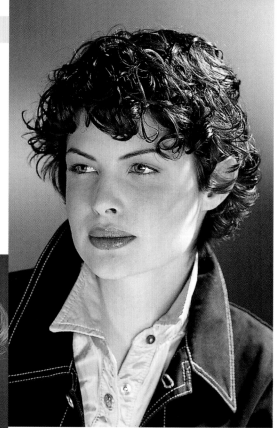

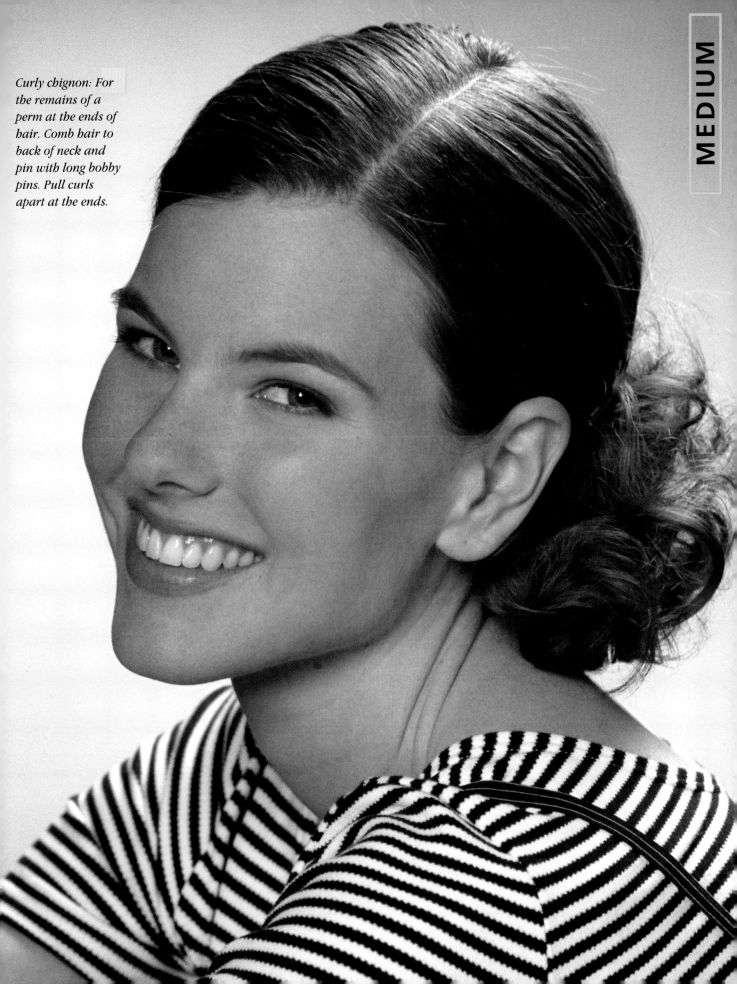

Curly chignon: For the remains of a perm at the ends of hair. Comb hair to back of neck and pin with long bobby pins. Pull curls apart at the ends.

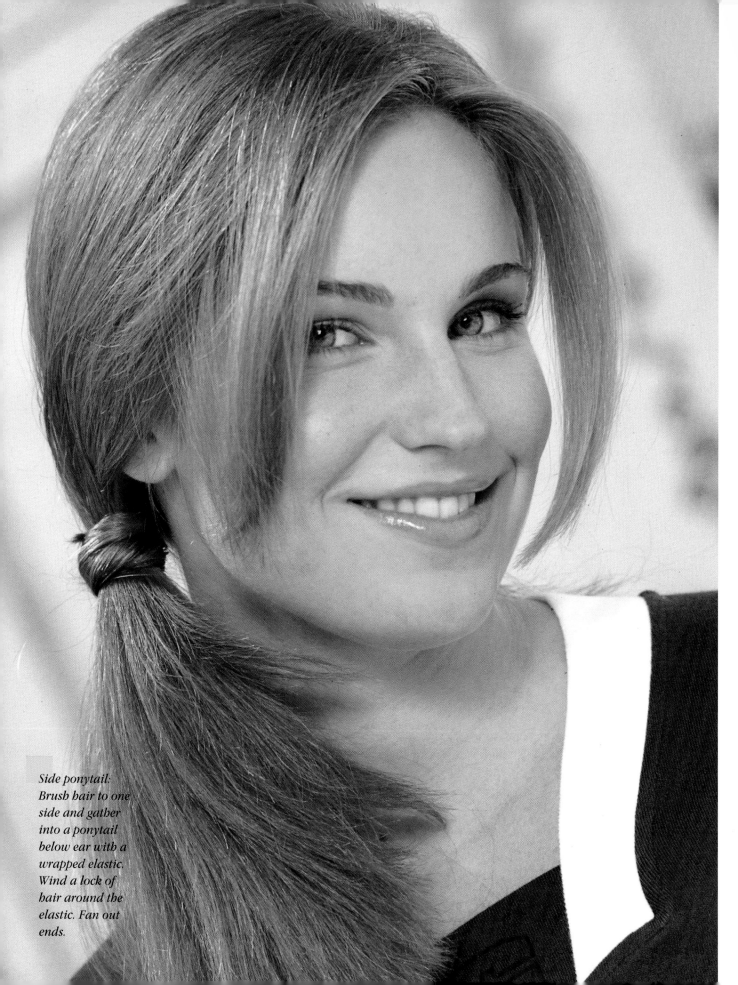

*Side ponytail:
Brush hair to one
side and gather
into a ponytail
below ear with a
wrapped elastic.
Wind a lock of
hair around the
elastic. Fan out
ends.*

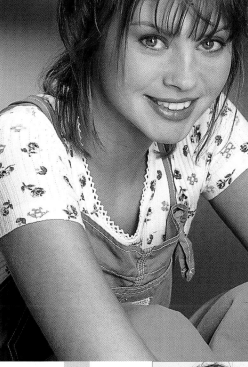

Feathered french roll: Roll hair into french roll (see pages 78–79), let ends stick out on top, and spread in a fan shape.

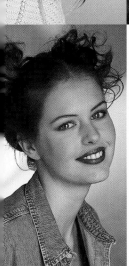

Twisted tails: Divide hair, tie into two tails. Each is again divided into two locks that are tightly wrapped around each other. Fold under and secure each with a pin behind the ear.

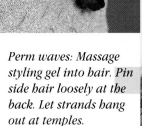

Perm waves: Massage styling gel into hair. Pin side hair loosely at the back. Let strands hang out at temples.

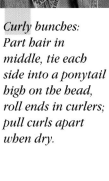

Curly bunches: Part hair in middle, tie each side into a ponytail high on the head, roll ends in curlers; pull curls apart when dry.

Tousled look: Hair of the lower layers remains free. The top layer is tied at the crown and then tousled; the ends are draped around.

Loosely knotted: To keep the sides from getting unkempt quickly, take the sides back and tie both into a loose knot; pin in place.

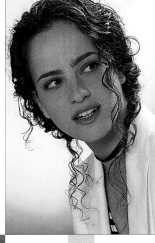

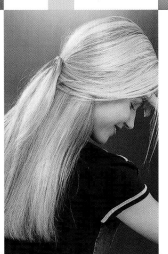

Country look: Permed hair is shaped into strands with styling gel. Braid hair at back, casually loose.

Hairband trick: Place a hairband in the hair as shown, and keep the back in place with a large, decorative comb.

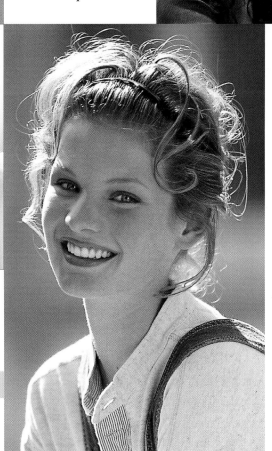

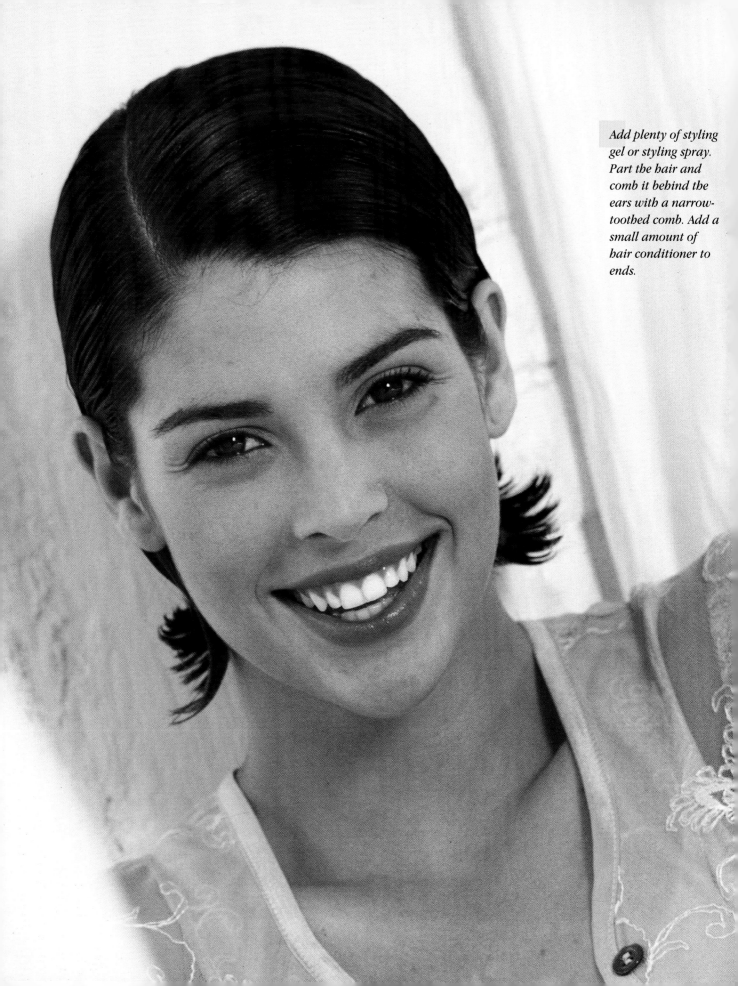

Add plenty of styling gel or styling spray. Part the hair and comb it behind the ears with a narrow-toothed comb. Add a small amount of hair conditioner to ends.

HIDE SPLIT ENDS: *quick styles*

Hide split ends in the top layer in a french roll. Comb styling liquid into the locks at the back and at the sides.

With shoulder length naturally wavy hair, split ends can easily be hidden by a ponytail with the ends turned under. Add styling gel first.

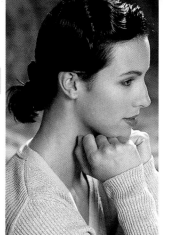

For naturally wavy hair, massage hair conditioner into the ends; use styling gel and comb the hair away from the face.

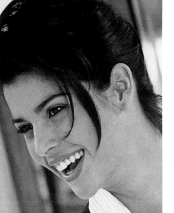

When it is mostly the top layer of the hair that is damaged, pull back and turn under at the back of the head; secure with bobby pins underneath.

If the ends of the top layer of hair are split, keep them off your face with a wide barrette or clasp. Smooth out the ends with styling liquid.

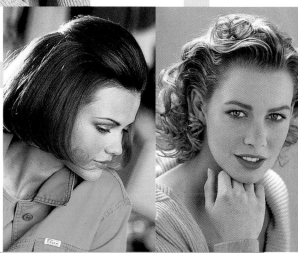

The best solution when the ends are split is a short haircut and lots of hair conditioning. The second-best solution: hairstyles that cleverly hide split ends.

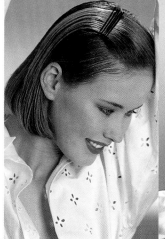

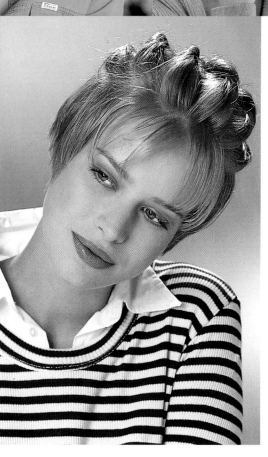

Twist locks of the top layer individually, turn under, and fasten with bobby pins.

Naturally wavy page-boy. Dampen hair with styling liquid; brush ends under in sections over the back of your hand.

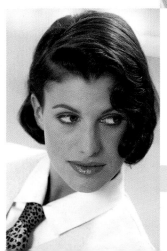

Split ends hide in a twisted chignon. Tie hair together at back, separate into individual locks, each finger width. Twist each one, let it curl up; pin in place.

Natural curls: Take one lock of hair from behind the ear and twist gently; pin in place at back of neck. Hair at the back is sectioned, twisted into loose locks, and pinned in place.

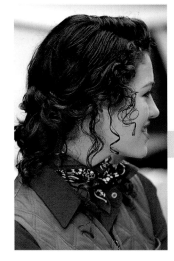

Pull hair back, comb back behind the ears, and secure with long clips. Ends are brushed under over the hand. Hold with hair spray.

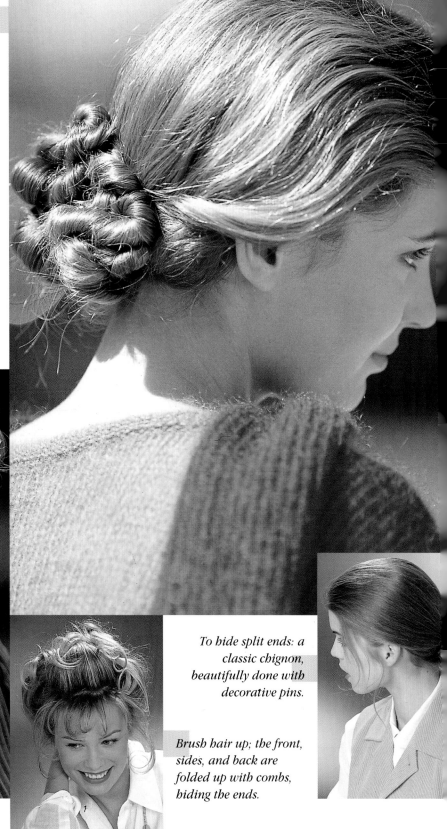

To hide split ends: a classic chignon, beautifully done with decorative pins.

Brush hair up; the front, sides, and back are folded up with combs, hiding the ends.

Hair is divided into small individual locks, wound up tight, and pinned around the head with hairpins. Add styling liquid first.

Dry hair on large rollers. Lightly tease at the roots. Fold in sections over the back of the hand, turn under, and secure with long pins.

Hair with a slight natural wave is tied together at the back. Twist into a chignon and secure with hairpins.

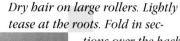

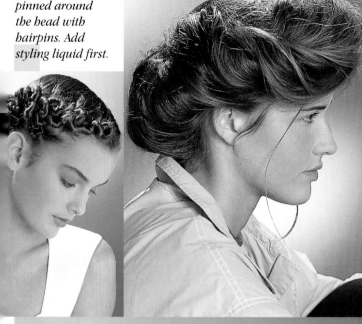

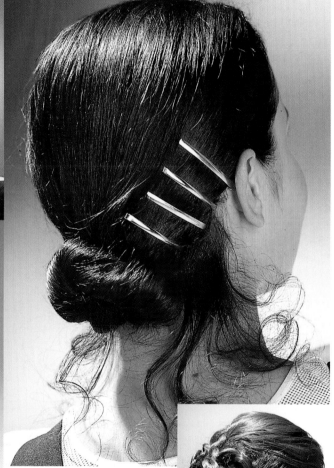

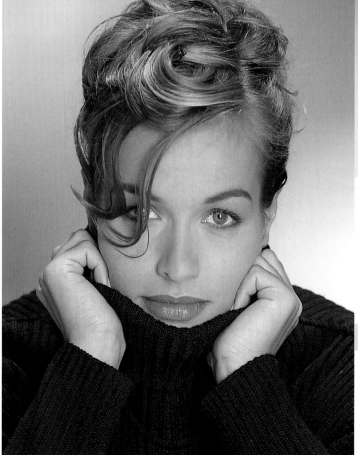

Tie hair in back in a ponytail; braid 10 minibraids; twist them into a snail shape. Pin with hairpins to hide ends.

Dry hair on velvet curlers, fold into french roll at back; pin in place. Arrange front in curls casually; pin some, let others hang free.

HELP! MY HAIR IS OILY!

Hair becomes oily very quickly because the sebaceous glands are sensitive to a hormone. Not much can be done about that. But with appropriate hair-care products and the right hairstyle, the problem can be controlled.

Tip 1: Shampoo your hair the correct way

Daily shampooing with a mild shampoo can keep the oil produced by the scalp from reaching the hair and making the hair look oily. Be sure to choose the correct shampoo: The right shampoo to use is one for normal hair. Such a shampoo contains active substances that are so mild that, even if used daily, they will not attack the hair or stimulate the scalp, which would produce even more oil. Shampoo for oily hair contains stronger substances; use it only if your hair has already become oily and is stringy.

Tip 2: The scalp is sensitive

The reason that too much oil is produced by the scalp is an innate sensitivity of the sebaceous glands to the hormone testosterone. This is most evident during puberty, but will get better over time. The basic fact is that cosmetic products can have very little effect on this situation. What can be prevented is the over-stimulation of the sebaceous glands, which could happen if you brush and comb too much, use too much heat during blow-drying, or use the wrong shampoo and water that is too hot when shampooing. A relaxing treatment for the scalp, applied for 10 minutes and then rinsed out before shampooing, is very beneficial. It relaxes the scalp and prevents dandruff. A scalp massage, applied to the scalp with the hair sectioned, also is very relaxing and calming.

Tip 3: Allow hair to air-dry naturally

An ideal haircut is one that needs neither blow-drying nor styling. It saves time and protects the scalp and hair ends. If there is not enough time to let hair air-dry naturally, a diffuser can be used, at least for partial drying. Bend your head down and massage the scalp as you blow-dry. This also adds volume.

Tip 4: Shampoo only the part of the hair that is close to the scalp

Shampooing the scalp alone is also a good solution to the problem of oily hair, but it is particularly good when the problem is an oily scalp. You need a small bottle with a nozzle (you probably can get one at the hair salon or store that sells hair products). Mix one part of shampoo for oily hair and four parts of warm water and apply directly to the dry scalp. Let the shampoo bubble up briefly, and then rinse. Whatever flows through the rest of the hair will be enough to clean it properly.

A perm can save you time and trouble if your hair becomes greasy too quickly, particularly when you have a haircut that can air-dry naturally. The additional advantage of a perm is that your hair will be more absorbent, because the hair surface has been chemically changed.

Tip 5: Keep hair standing up straight at the roots

All styling tricks that keep your hair from lying flat on the head are useful, including gently teasing and spraying the roots with styling spray, applied with the head bent down. When blow-drying, be sure that the air flows away from the scalp and the sebaceous glands. Apply volumizing setting mousse.

HELP! SPLIT ENDS!

Hair that feels rough to the touch has small holes on the surface. Moisture from inside the hair shaft can evaporate, and hair substance has been lost. Giving your hair special care can at least conceal this loss, as described in the following tips.

Tip 1: Have the ends cut regularly

Hair will immediately look healthier and more cared for, and will flow more beautifully when the frizzy ends are removed. It does not need to be cut short. It is usually sufficient to remove a few millimeters to get a healthier look. However, small brush-like ends may be a sign that the inside of the hair shafts are split, sometimes as much as a few centimeters (an inch). If too little is cut, the ends may quickly split again. A one-time radical cut, from which the hair will grow out in better condition, usually gives the best results.

Tip 2: Splice-cut for split ends

People with long hair and many split ends who simply can't decide to have their hair cut may ask for what is called a splice cut, in which not only the damaged ends of the lower layers are cut, but also the usually somewhat shorter and particularly badly damaged top layers. When a splice cut is done, the hair is separated into thin locks and tightly turned around itself; the ends that stick out are trimmed off with a sharp pair of scissors.

Tip 3: Replace keratin loss as much as possible

Special products for stressed hair include substances similar to the keratin naturally present in hair. Filling microscopically fine holes in the hair shaft makes hair smooth and easy to handle again. In addition, these preparations prevent split ends, because the substances they contain envelop the ends and prevent splitting. For heavily stressed hair, apply an intensive treatment lotion after each shampooing, one designed especially for stressed hair. Once the hair is again flexible and firm, one treatment every fourth shampooing will suffice.

Absolutely taboo for stressed hair and split ends: anything that roughens the surface of the hair shaft or punctures it or scrapes it. Rollers with brushes inside, brushes with plastic bristles that are not smooth, and cheap combs also are forbidden. The following also are bad for hair whose keratin structure has been damaged: heat and overstretching when wet, which happens when hair is wrapped over a brush and hot-air dried. Use curling irons and heated curlers sparingly.

Tip 4: Avoid perms with drastic hair color changes

In both perms and hair color changes, the hair structure is chemically loosened so that the desired changes of style or pigment can take place. It's much safer to perm and color separately; coloring healthy hair makes the results much more brilliant, and doing a perm separately will result in its looking more natural and beautiful. You risk injuring your hair badly if you do both together.

Tip 5: Conceal hair damage by using some styling tricks

Coarse hair and damaged ends will be less noticeable if you decide on the wet or gel look. Instead of stressing your hair with daily blow-drying, comb your hair through with styling gel, styling liquid, or mousse. You will find many such style suggestions in this book.

CHAPTER III

Evening styles FOR

On the next pages are styling
suggestions for a glamorous look,
some for every hair length. You'll also
find instructions for creating a french roll,
a french braid, or waves in the style of a
1940s movie star, as well
as many hairstyles
with curls.

A STARRING ROLE

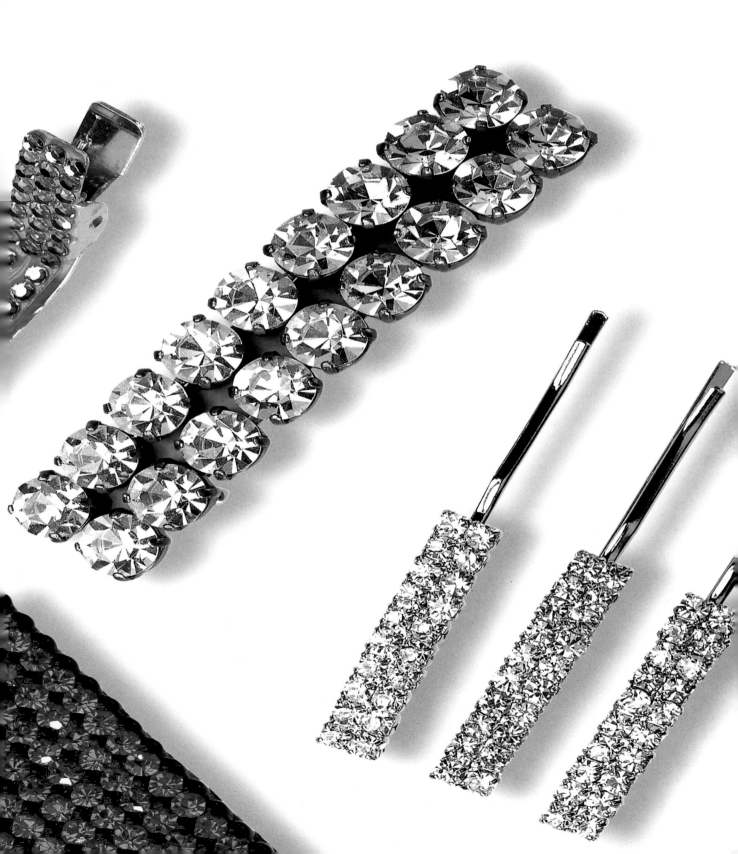

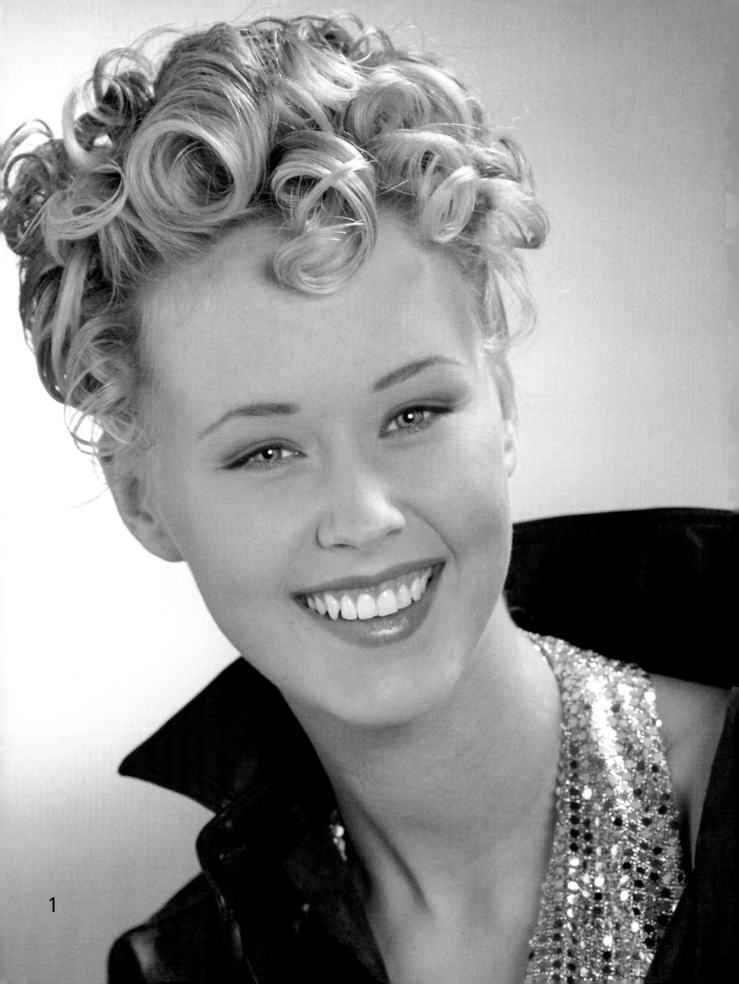

1

SHORT *evening styles*

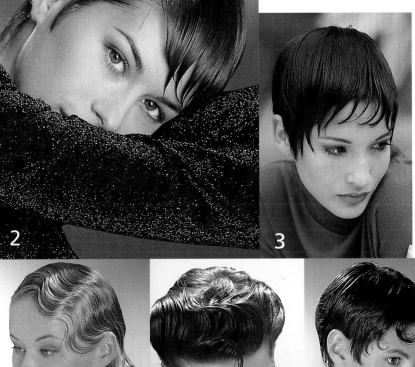

1 *Curls: Apply light styling spray to dry hair. With a thick curling iron, create curls on top of head. Do not comb out!*
2 *Wet look: Part hair on side, comb behind ear on short side; on the other side, pull the hair diagonally onto the forehead. Apply styling gel or gel wax beforehand to damp hair. Use styling gel on damp hair for all the following:* **3** *End work: Pull the ends above forehead forward into distinct bangs and spray with hair spray.* **4** *Making waves: Part hair on side; with side of hand, push the hair into waves.* **5** *Elvis style: Natural waves. Grab hair on top of head, pull back, then push together and back towards face. Comb sides up.* **6** *Sideburns: Add styling gel, form half-round curls at the temples and on the forehead.* **7** *Temple waves: Part hair on side; form waves on the wide side.* **8** *Natural waves: Shape waves in parallel lines from front to back with clips, and dry hair with a diffuser.*

Clever styling tricks provide a festive touch, not only for long hair. Short and medium-length hair also can look very sophisticated for a night out.

1 *Ballerina chignon: Add styling gel to damp hair. Create a large wave with a comb in front of each ear. Pull hair back, twist in a knot, and secure at the neck.* **2** *1950s style: Tease hair at crown. Curl hair with a curling iron up to ear height. Tie top layer together at the back, turn under, and secure.* **3** *Mini braids: Make thin braids on either side of the part; secure the ends with styling lacquer. With a curling iron, gently turn the ends under.* **4** *Spiral look: Dampen hair with setting lotion, roll hair on curlers placed vertically. Remove curlers and simply shake hair out.* **5** *Corkscrew curls: Apply setting lotion, roll hair to the roots, one lock at a time, on a curling iron. Clip in place and let hair cool down; do not comb out.* **6** *Romantic: Naturally slightly wavy hair is curled with a curling iron, and the curls fastened on top of the head.* **7** *Ready for the movies: A straight bob with hair parted low. Using styling liquid, comb hair behind ears and away from forehead. Lift bangs up and hold in place with styling spray.*

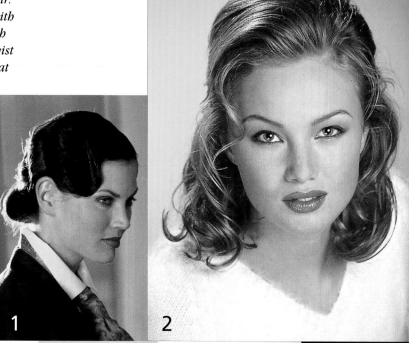

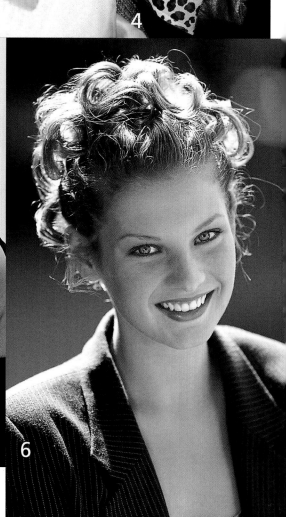

MEDIUM

MEDIUM LENGTH *evening styles*

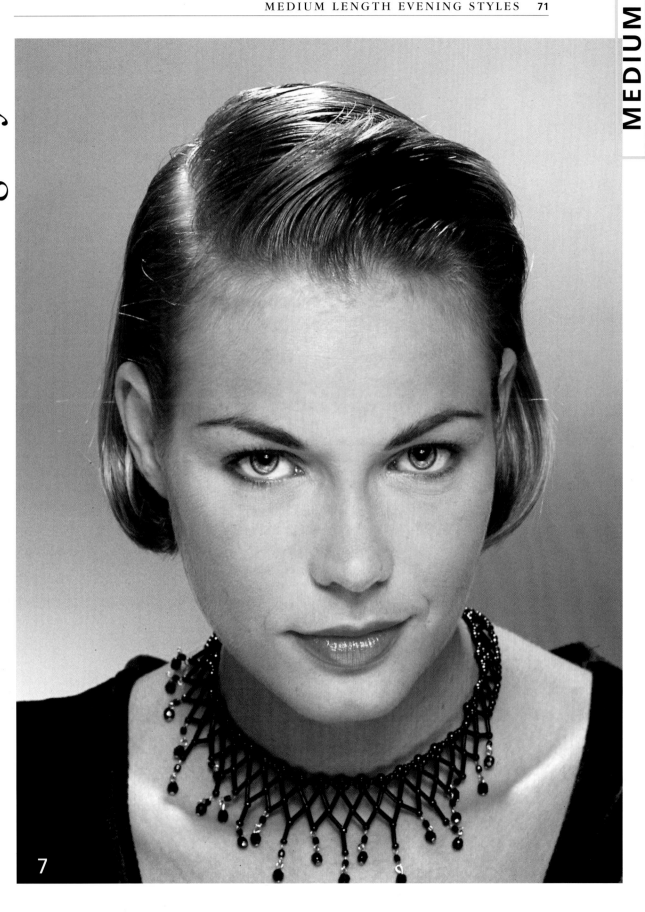

7

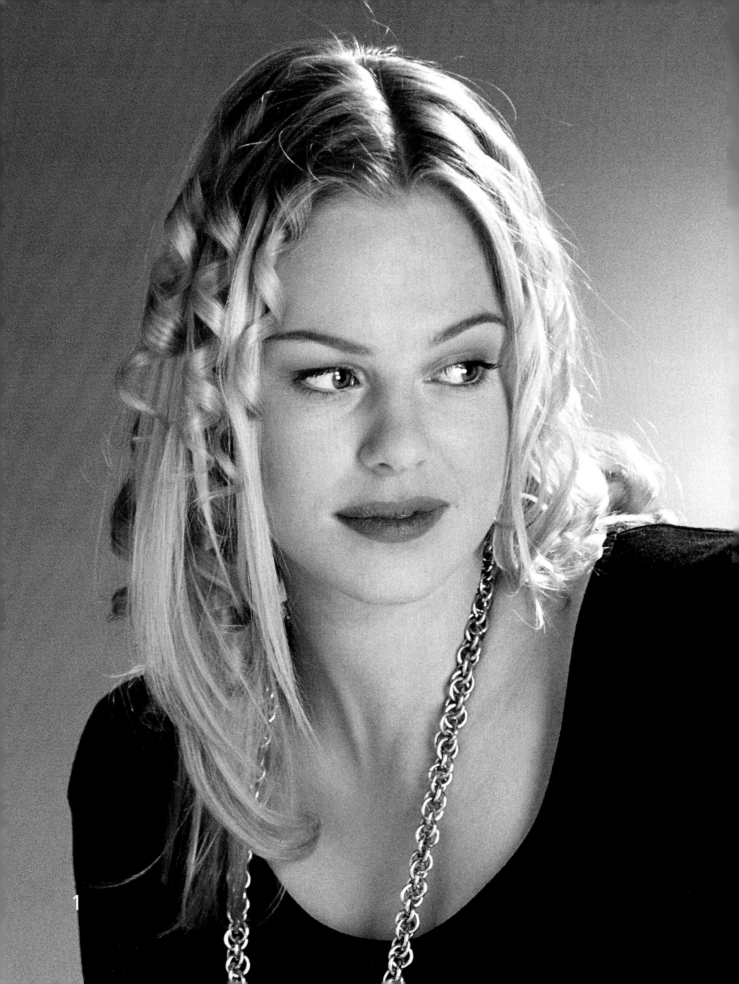

LONG *evening styles*

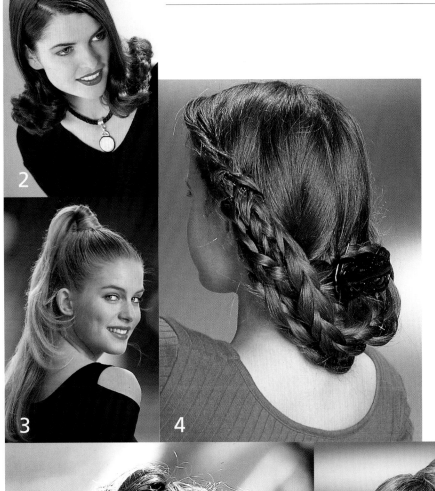

1 *Spiral curls: Blow-dry hair straight. Take a few locks on each side of a middle part and curl halfway up with a curling iron. Keep curled until the hair cools; then apply styling spray.* **2** *Curling up: Apply styling gel; make a divided part. Bend the ends out and up with a large curling iron. Each curl must be clipped in place to cool. Hold with styling lacquer.* **3** *Barbie style: Pull the hair up tightly at the highest point of the crown into a pony-tail. One lock of hair is wrapped around the elastic.* **4** *Beautifully braided: Starting at the temple, make two braids on each side. Loop them at the back and secure the ends with a barrette.* **5** *Hair tower: Tie the hair in a ponytail at the top of the head, wind the length of the hair around the base, and pull up a bit. Fasten well.* **6** *Pin curls: Roll the hair on warm curlers. When the hair has cooled down, remove the curlers and twist each curl around two fingers. Fasten at the top of the head. Pull a few strands out of the curls to hang in front of and behind the ears.*

7 *1940s look: Starting at the temple, take one lock and twist it towards the back, adding other locks one at a time as you move backwards. At the back, fold both twists up and secure with rhinestone barrettes.*
8 *Coiled: Roll hair on heated rollers. When hair is cool, shake curls out and tie a ponytail at the top of the head. Braid one small lock and tie it around the base of the ponytail.* **9** *Knotted: Casually pull your hair back. Divide hair into an upper and lower section at the back of your head. Tie a knot with both locks and secure ends.*
10 *Zigzag curls: Apply setting lotion to damp hair. One lock at a time, wind hair around the ends of a giant hairpin in crisscross pattern. (You can make large hairpins of stiff wire.) Dry with diffuser. Let hair cool. Curls are not combed out, just sprayed with setting lotion. Twist a few locks on the top of the head, let them curl loosely, and pin in place.*
11 *Super twist: Bind hair together with an elastic low at the neck. Create a vertical opening above the elastic and flip the tail up and through the opening.*

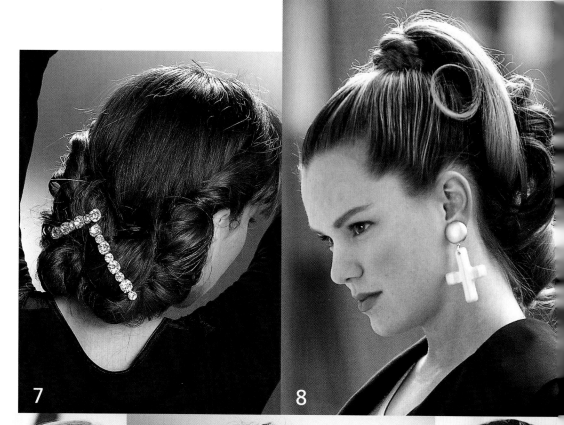

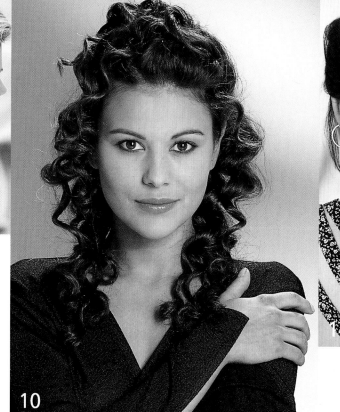

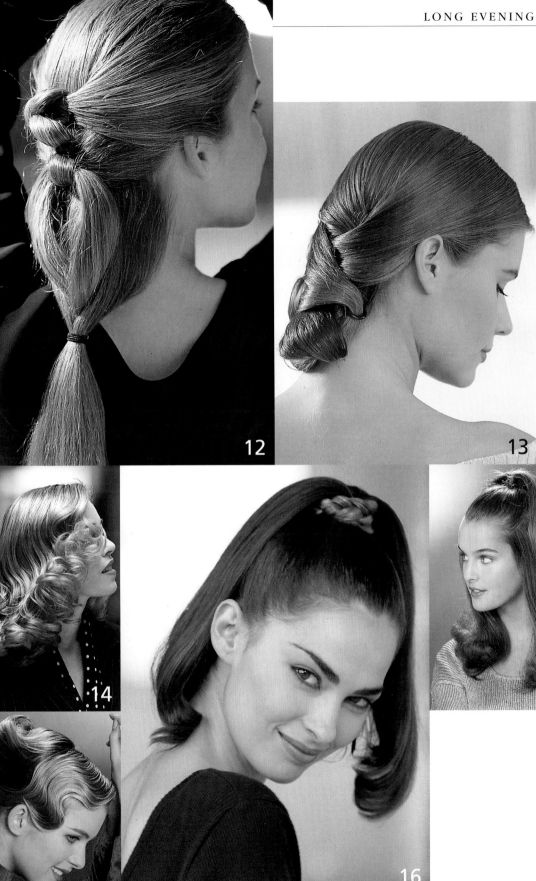

12 *Double knot: Take two sections of hair from the temples and knot together in the back. Take a section on each side from underneath the temple hair and tie into another knot. Bind the hair below the second knot together with the rest of the hair below it with an elastic.*
13 *Braiding: Apply styling liquid. At the back of the head, halfway down, braid hair in a french braid (see page 80). Turn ends under and pin well.* **14** *Fabulous waves: Apply styling lotion. Roll lower third of the hair on medium-size curlers; clip and hold curls in place vertically. Use a wide-tooth comb to comb out. Important: hair must be angle-cut.* **15** *Glamour: Part hair on side; turn hair at the back into a french roll (see page 79), apply styling gel to the front, and push hair into a large wave.* **16** *Lolita look: Twist a synthetic hair braid around the base of a ponytail; blow-dry the ends, turning them inside.* **17** *Barbie style: Hair in front is brushed back tightly, tied in a ponytail, and fanned out.*

1 *Hippie mane: Divide the hair in finger-thick locks, roll on curlers, but leave the parts near the scalp unrolled. Comb hair with your fingers only.*
2 *Romantic: Starting near the center part, braid hair loosely. Join at the back with a barrette. Pull small strands out of the braid to create a wispy veil all around.* **3** *Twisted chignon: Tie hair together at the back. Take finger-thick locks one at a time, twist each around itself, and tie into a thick chignon at the base of the neck.* **4** *Pin-up curls: Enhance your natural curls by rolling on curlers. When dry, pin each one on top of your head.*
5 *Lazybones: Tie the hair loosely together on top and decorate with a small ribbon.* **6** *Tamed: Lift the hair up in front with spread-out fingers, pushing slightly forward to create a domed shape, and pin it so the part near the head curves out.* **7** *Movie-star curls: Apply styling gel and comb hair flat. Starting at ear height, curl hair—one lock at a time—with a thick curling iron.* **8** *A mop of curls: Masses of locks fall over the edge of a zigzag hair comb, which is pushed into the hair from the neck up towards the back of the head.*

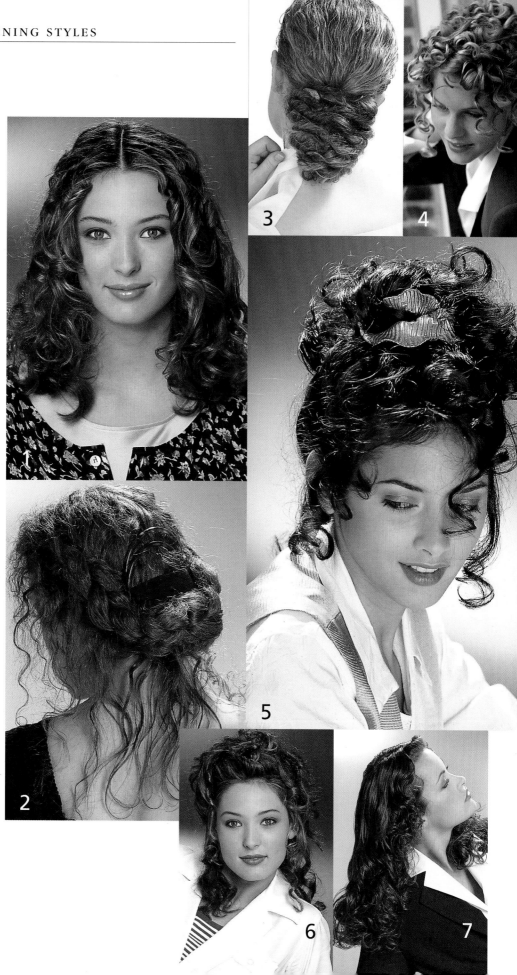

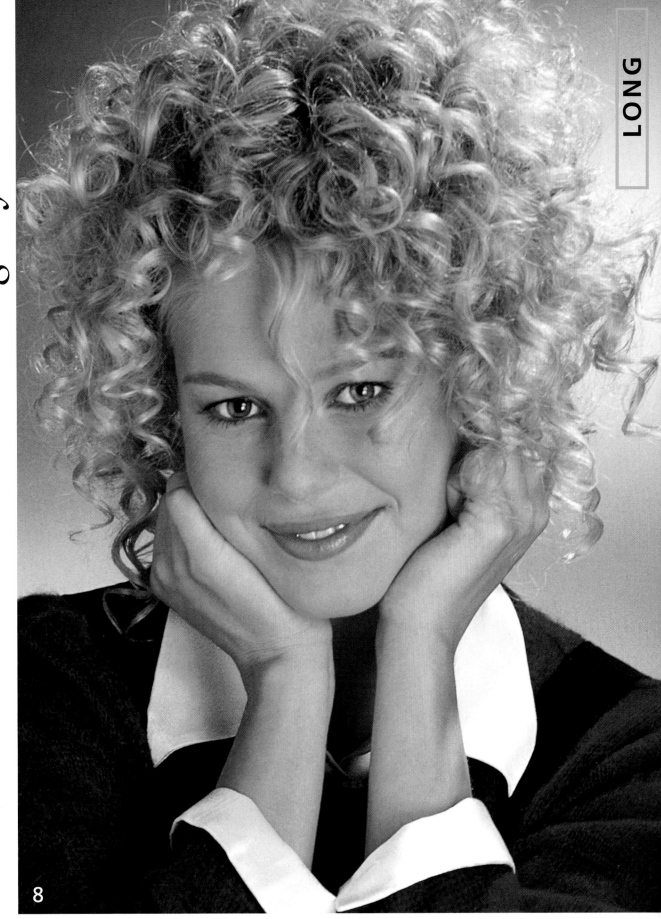

LONG CURLY *evening styles*

8

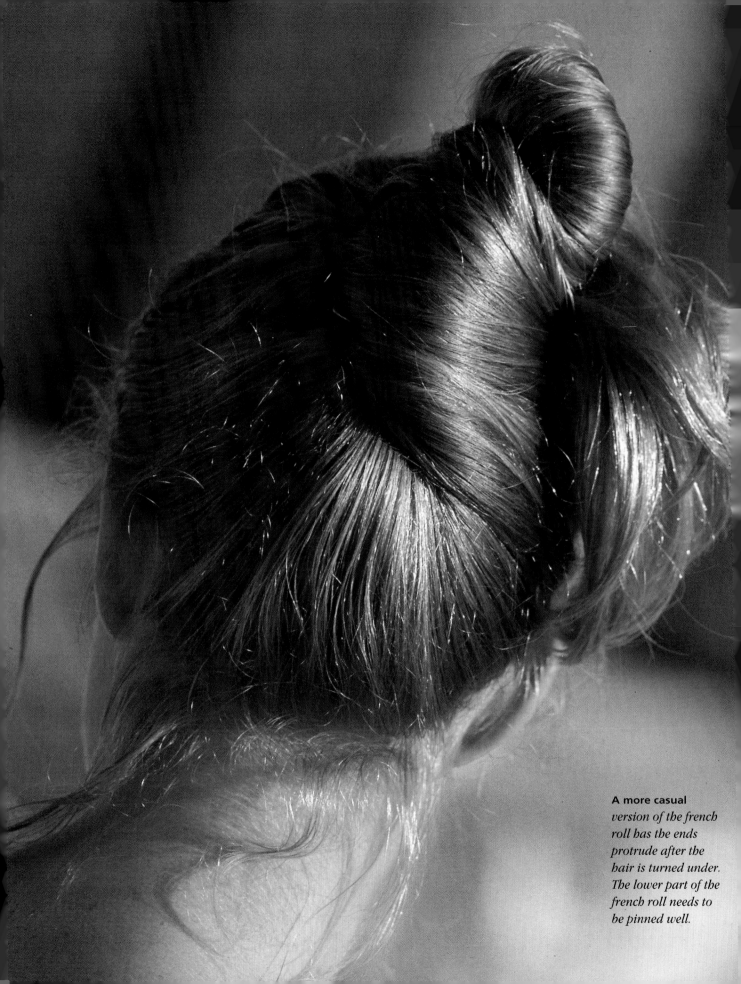

A more casual
version of the french
roll has the ends
protrude after the
hair is turned under.
The lower part of the
french roll needs to
be pinned well.

CLASSIC *french roll*

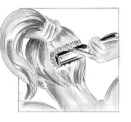

Brush hair up to the crown. With your left hand, hold hair together one-third up the length

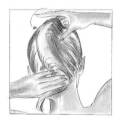

Turn all hair under near the scalp around the middle finger of the right hand

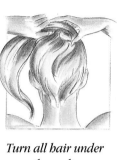

Turn the ends underneath on themselves into a roll and pin

EXTRA TIP: Hair becomes easier to handle when volumizing mousse or lotion for blow-drying is used.

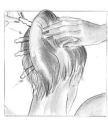

Pin the roll through the center to your head with a long clip, from top down. Hold with hairpins

Hair for the french roll, french braid (page 80), chignon (page 83), and movie-star waves (page 84) must be at least shoulder length, preferably unlayered. Hair may be straight or curly; bangs are okay.

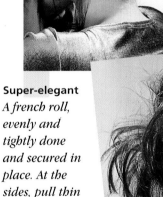

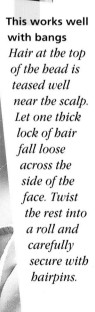

Super-elegant
A french roll, evenly and tightly done and secured in place. At the sides, pull thin strands out of the roll and shape with hair wax.

Casual variation for wavy hair
Front hair is not totally smooth. Important: when combing out, add volume at top of the head. Pin roll loosely. Tousle bangs with mousse.

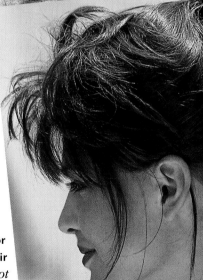

This works well with bangs
Hair at the top of the head is teased well near the scalp. Let one thick lock of hair fall loose across the side of the face. Twist the rest into a roll and carefully secure with hairpins.

CLASSIC *french braid*

A modern *interpreation: separate the top layer and tease well from below to get good volume at the top of the head. Finish by adding a barrette or tie at the base of the braid.*

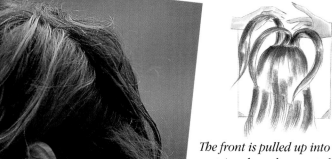

Wide and short
also looks good. Make a french braid with loose lines; fold braid in half and pin under. Pull thin locks loose from the sides of the braid.

The front is pulled up into a triangle and separated into 3 equal parts. Drop the middle portion and make two normal braid turns with the outer two parts

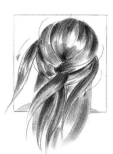

Alternating left and right, lift one lock with thumb from rest of hair; add into top lock of braid. Make one braid turn; then add more hair

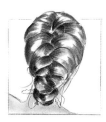

When all hair on the sides is added, continue braiding normally and secure the ends well; turn ends under and pin in place, if desired

EXTRA TIP:
Braid hair while it's damp and go to sleep. The next morning, your hair will be magnificently wavy.

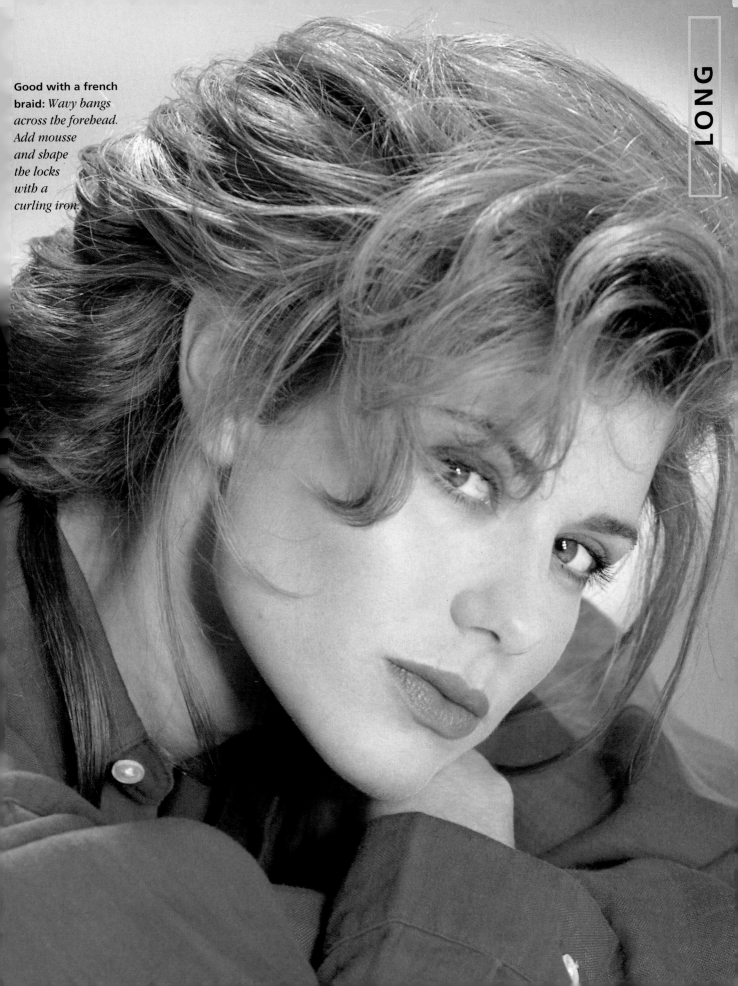

Good with a french braid: *Wavy bangs across the forehead. Add mousse and shape the locks with a curling iron.*

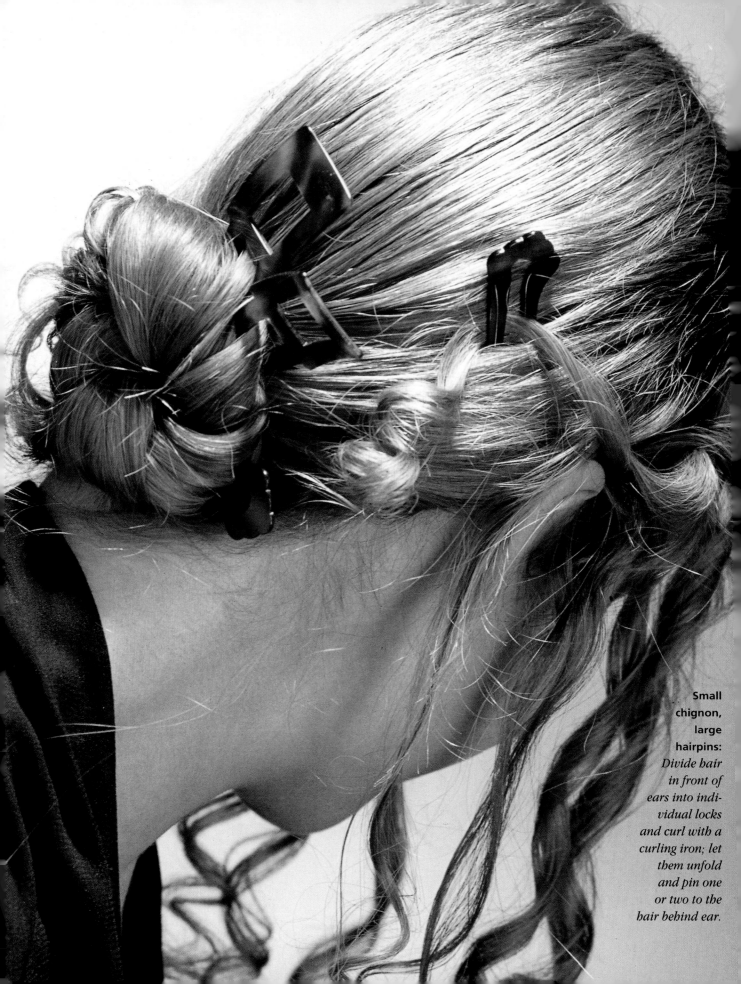

Small chignon, large hairpins: *Divide hair in front of ears into individual locks and curl with a curling iron; let them unfold and pin one or two to the hair behind ear.*

CLASSIC *chignon*

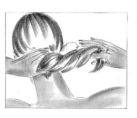

Brush hair back firmly, hold at back of neck, and with the other hand tightly twist it around itself to create tension...

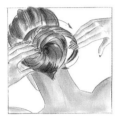

...letting the chignon almost shape itself. Hold the chignon at the center with the index finger of the left hand and wind the rest of hair around

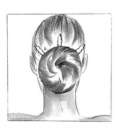

Carefully push the ends under the chignon and fasten with pins

EXTRA TIP: For a tighter fit, push hairpins at an angle into the chignon; then flatten them against your scalp, sliding them in place under the chignon.

Double chignon: *Comb hair back tightly with a lot of styling gel. Tie together in back at neck; then separate in two. Twist each half into a loop. Fan out each loop with your fingers and fasten.*

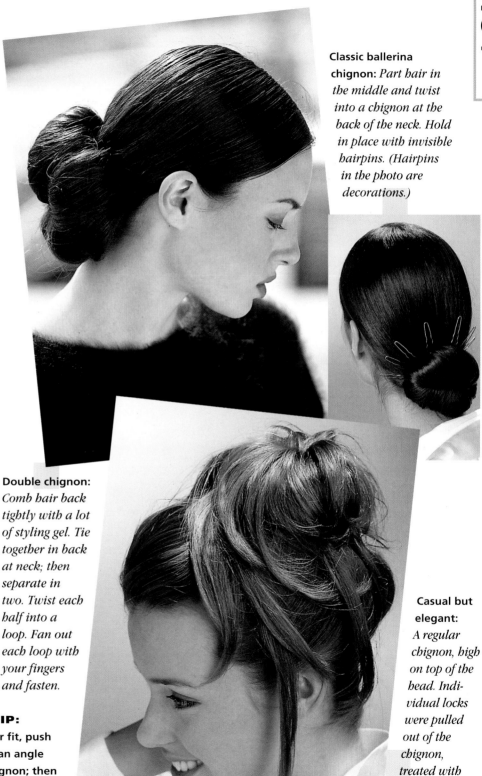

Classic ballerina chignon: *Part hair in the middle and twist into a chignon at the back of the neck. Hold in place with invisible hairpins. (Hairpins in the photo are decorations.)*

Casual but elegant: *A regular chignon, high on top of the head. Individual locks were pulled out of the chignon, treated with gel, and arranged decoratively on one side.*

For the big soft wave in front *hair must be slightly layered. Part hair on the side; roll in curlers on both sides, starting at the part. The base is teased and held with hair spray.*

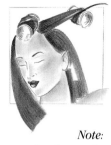

Note: Start by placing the roller in the middle of a lock of hair; smooth ends around the roller. Only then, finish rolling hair up to scalp. Clip rollers in place

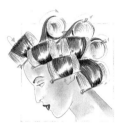

Side view: One roller at the top of head, with two behind it rolled towards the back. One each to left and right of the part, one under at each temple, and two smaller ones above each ear

When hair is very long *only the ends will hold a wave. But that can be beautiful. Blow-dry ends over a round brush; leave it in place until hair is completely cool. Hold with hair spray.*

Back view: one roller is set into gap on each side of the back. Hair left in the middle underneath and on the sides is rolled on smaller curlers

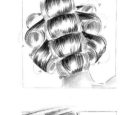

Remove rollers after half an hour. Brush hair from the back forward, one lock at a time, and shape it into large waves with a brush over the back of hand

Movie-star waves *in a slightly layered long mane. Shape ends with a round brush, held vertically. Hold with styling lacquer.*

EXTRA TIP: Dampen hair with styling lotion, roll on heated or self-stick rollers. Let cool or dry well.

CLASSIC movie-star waves

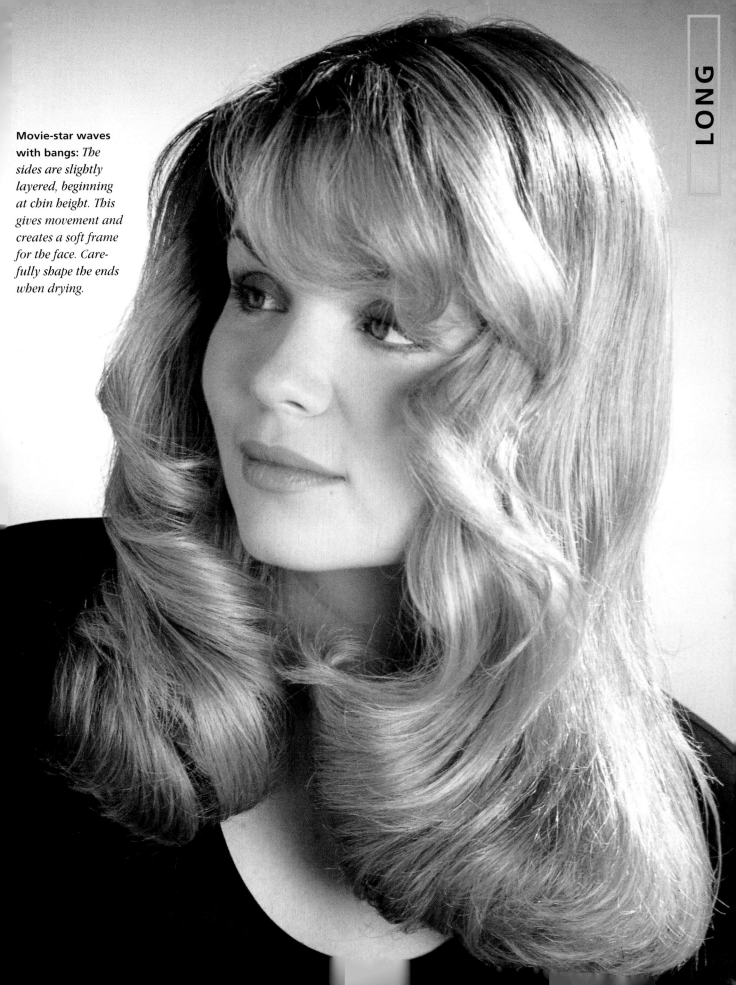

Movie-star waves with bangs: *The sides are slightly layered, beginning at chin height. This gives movement and creates a soft frame for the face. Carefully shape the ends when drying.*

A BEAUTIFUL PERM...

A permanent wave gives hair body, substance, and movement. It saves time and work when styling. Many factors are involved if a perm is to turn out the way you had hoped and last as long as you want it to, as described below.

Factor 1: Determine beforehand with a professional what is possible

Don't try perming your own hair. Perms involve chemicals, timing, and expertise that you don't have. Insist on a thorough consultation if it is your first perm. Your hairstylist needs to know what you expect. You need to know if what you want can be accomplished, given your hair type. No one can give a 100% guarantee of the outcome anyhow, but try to minimize unpleasant surprises. The following should be decided beforehand:

◆ Is your hair to get more body overall? Or only near the scalp? Or do you only want to give your hair more movement in a certain place—for instance, in front?
◆ Do you want the curls to be small and tousled, so you can let your hair air-dry naturally...
◆ ...or do you want to keep your present hairstyle and use the perm only as a foundation to keep your hair in better shape?

Here are some suggestions: Show your hairstylist photos of hairstyles you like. If the stylist discourages you from trying one because the quality of your hair is not right for a particular hair-style, compromise. It doesn't pay to push for a result that can't be guaranteed. Remember, if the curls turn out badly, you'll have to either cut them off or let them grow out.

Factor 2: Treat your new curls properly

Freshly permed hair is sensitive. A perm will last longer when it has been given two or three days to settle. This means: waiting at least two days until shampooing the hair. And under no circumstances should either a brush, rollers, hair dryer, or curling iron be used. The structure of each individual hair has been loosened, and all the above would unnecessarily stretch the curls, causing them to quickly lose their resilience. Don't color and perm at the same time.

Factor 3: Permed hair needs good care

Even the best perm changes the natural structure of the hair. This means the surface of each individual hair becomes rough. Therefore, use a conditioner or acid rinse after each shampooing. A conditioning treatment now and then also is helpful. This also affects the elasticity of the curls.

Factor 4: Newly permed hair needs to be cut frequently

Very important: Have the ends cut no later than four weeks after the perm. This creates new tension and prevents split ends or harsh-looking curls. Limp curls can be given new pep by applying a moisturizing lotion to damp hair. Each conditioning rinse or treatment also improves the tension of the curls.

Factor 5: A perm must be properly styled

Permed curls turn out best when allowed to air-dry naturally. Spray damp hair with moisturizing lotion, bend over, and massage hair with your fingers until it dries. If you are in a hurry, a diffuser should be used, since the airflow comes out of many small jets and is gentler than a dryer without a diffuser. When hair is almost dry, tousle it with all ten fingers until completely cool.

...SUPER COLOR

It's true for hair color, just as for clothing and makeup: for a color to make you more beautiful or keep you looking beautiful, it must go with your own color harmony. For that reason, it's important to determine what that harmony is.

Color Tip 1: Find out your color type

Your color harmony or type is the result of the natural pigmentation of your eyes, skin, and hair. Roughly speaking, there are two kinds: the warm and the cold. The warm color harmonies (spring and fall types) are people whose natural coloring is sunny, with a yellow-gold-orange base. The cold color harmonies mean blue-silvery colors (people with this coloring are the summer and winter types). You should determine your color type and always stay with either the warm or the cold shades, depending on which your natural color harmonies are. Then you can change your hair color but still end up with pleasing results.

Color Tip 2: Hold a sample lock of dyed hair up to your face

By now, many beauty salons have color charts in which a variety of hair samples are divided into cold and warm shades. It is not sufficient to simply look at them. Hold the sample of the color you have chosen against your face in the area of your eyes or, if that is too difficult, at least against the back of your hand. Only in this way will you be able to determine if the new shade truly harmonizes with the natural coloring of your body.

Rule of thumb for choosing a color: For the summer type: ashen and silver hair shades. For the winter type: blue-black, peroxide blond, bluish burgundy red, or dark hazelnut brown. The spring type can choose almost any shade that is gold-blonde or honey brown. The fall type should stay with warm copper and rust tones.

Color Tip 3: Test a color first with tinting mousse

If you are not sure about your choice, run a test first with tinting mousse to see how a new color harmonizes with your complexion and eye color. If the color is correct, you can proceed with a more permanent product. If the color is still not quite right, the hairstylist can mix a specific shade for you.

Color Tip 4: Leave drastic color changes to the professional hairstylist

If you're thinking of making a drastic color change (which you should think about very carefully because it is very stressful to the hair), the experience of a professional is absolutely necessary. If you are making a big change in hair color, the roots need to be treated properly and the ends need to be cut regularly if you want the color to be even and look natural. This is particularly important with long hair, which often has porous ends that need techniques that are only available to a professional. Coloring agents penetrate porous hair much faster than they penetrate unprocessed hair, and they also are washed out much faster. It takes experience and a sensitive touch to determine how long a coloring agent should be left on the various parts of your hair.

Color Tip 5: Use color reflex shampoo at home

This shampoo is a mix of three-fourths regular shampoo and one-fourth tinting emulsion. It can be mixed specifically for your hair color. A basic recommendation: use test-mousse (see Tip 3) and hair coloring preparations made by the same company. This helps ensure that your hair color will remain the same.

Color Tip 6: Don't perm and color at the same time

Wait a few weeks between these processes; even so, by doing both, you are risking injuring your hair.

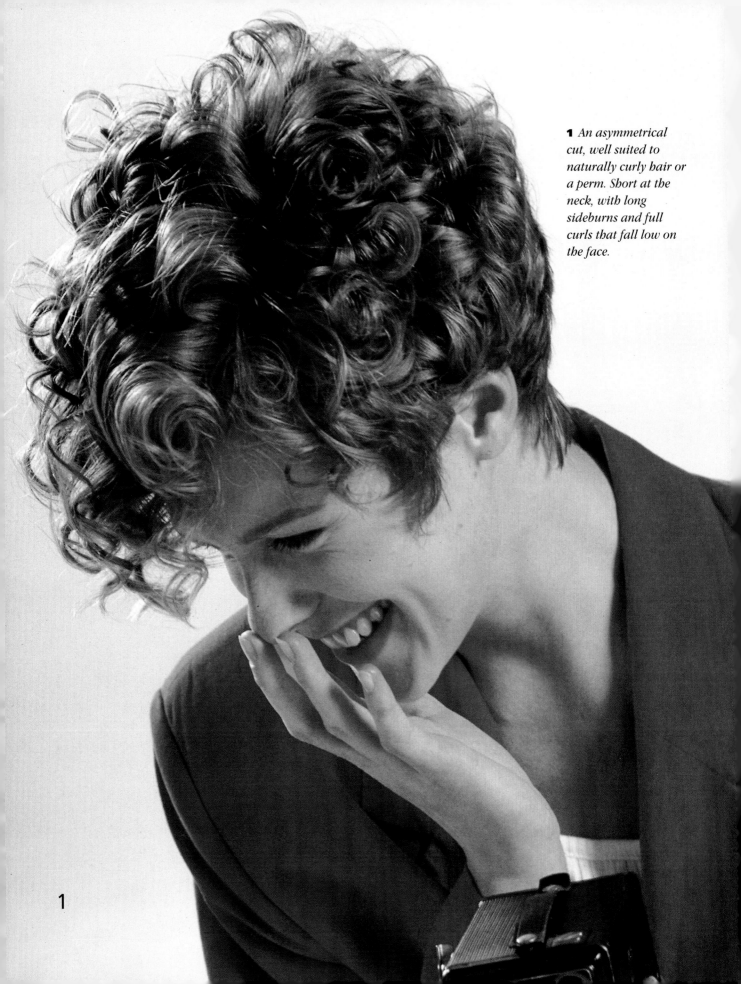

1 *An asymmetrical cut, well suited to naturally curly hair or a perm. Short at the neck, with long sideburns and full curls that fall low on the face.*

1

SHORT CURLY *styles*

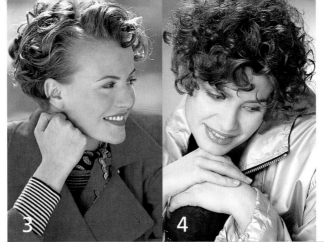

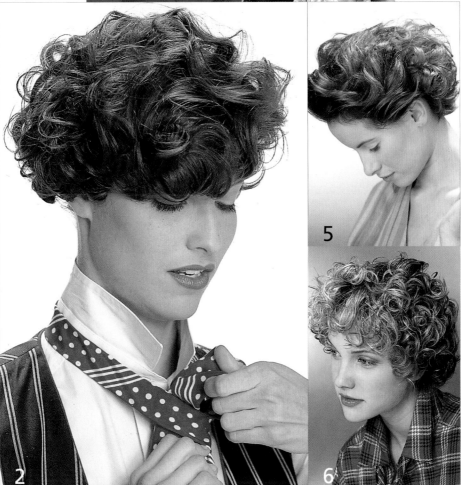

3 *The basic cut is a bob: Dampen with styling gel and comb behind the ear on one side.* **4** *A mop of curls with a short layered cut that has a long top layer. This can also be done with curlers.* **5** *Naturally wavy or permed, layered towards the back and blow-dried with the head turned down for added body.* **6** *Curler-made curls on a well-layered mushroom cut. The curls will last longer when they are sprayed with light styling spray and then curled with a thin curling iron. Hold the curling iron vertically when wrapping the curls.* **7** *Well-layered naturally wavy hair; add volumizing mousse and blow-dry the front, pulling the hair up with your fingers.*

2 *Short pageboy, created with heated curlers, is fluffed up, then held with styling spray.*

People with natural curls are lucky; others can get the same effect with a perm, rollers, or curlers. Curls are always flattering and make almost anybody look beautiful, regardless of how long their hair is.

1 *Perm with small curls on a bob cut without bangs. After shampooing, spray them with moisturizing lotion and let air-dry naturally.*

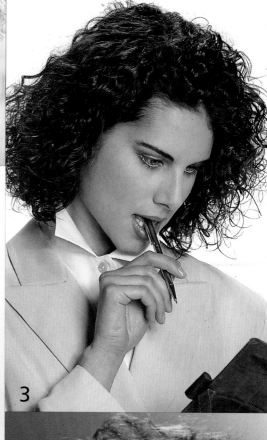

2 *For special occasions: baroque curls. Spray the naturally wavy or permed hair with styling lotion, and use a curling iron, one lock at a time. Secure curls with clips until cold. Use only your fingers to tousle hair.*
3 *Perm with small curls, wet look. Massage styling liquid into the hair and let air-dry naturally. In front, twist one lock into a mini knot and pin.*
4 *Corkscrew curls: Not for every day, but well worth the effort for a special occasion. The shoulder-length blunt-cut hair is separated into not-too-thin locks and curled with a curling iron from the ends up to temple height, with the iron turned vertically. Clip in place and let cool well, and apply styling spray. When dry, use fingers only to arrange hair.* **5** *Curly look: Naturally wavy hair is curled with a curling iron; curls are not combed out, only shaped with styling gel. Fasten a handful of curls loosely on top of head.* **6** *Roll hair up on heated curlers; when cool, massage hair with fingers, apply styling gel to ends, and twist.*

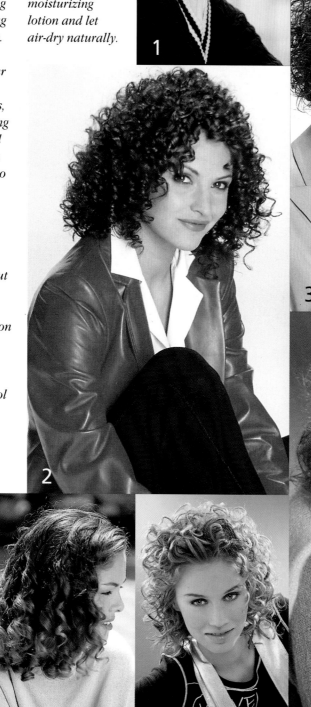

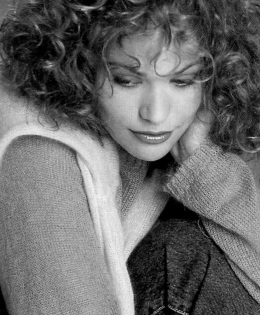

MEDIUM

MEDIUM LENGTH *curly styles*

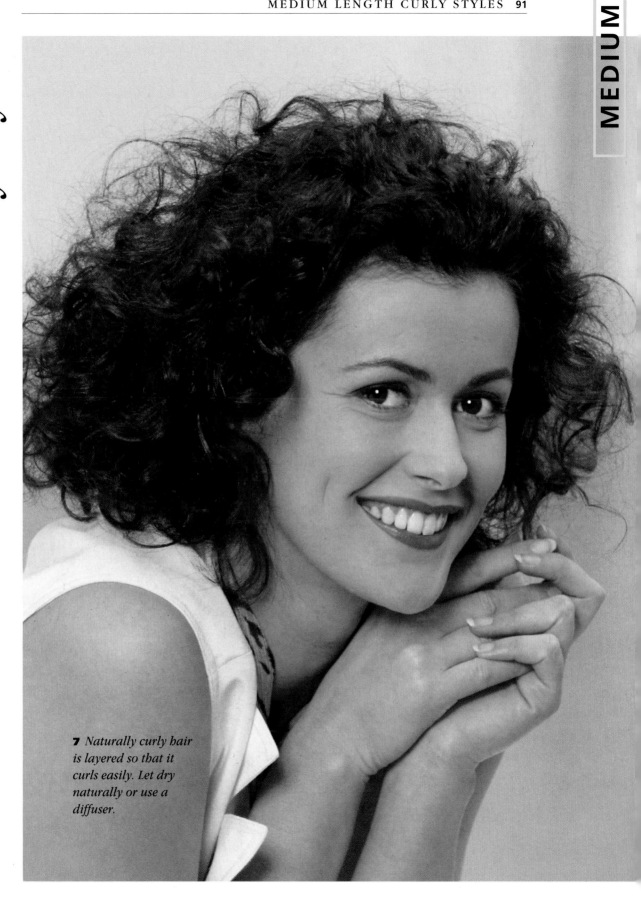

7 *Naturally curly hair is layered so that it curls easily. Let dry naturally or use a diffuser.*

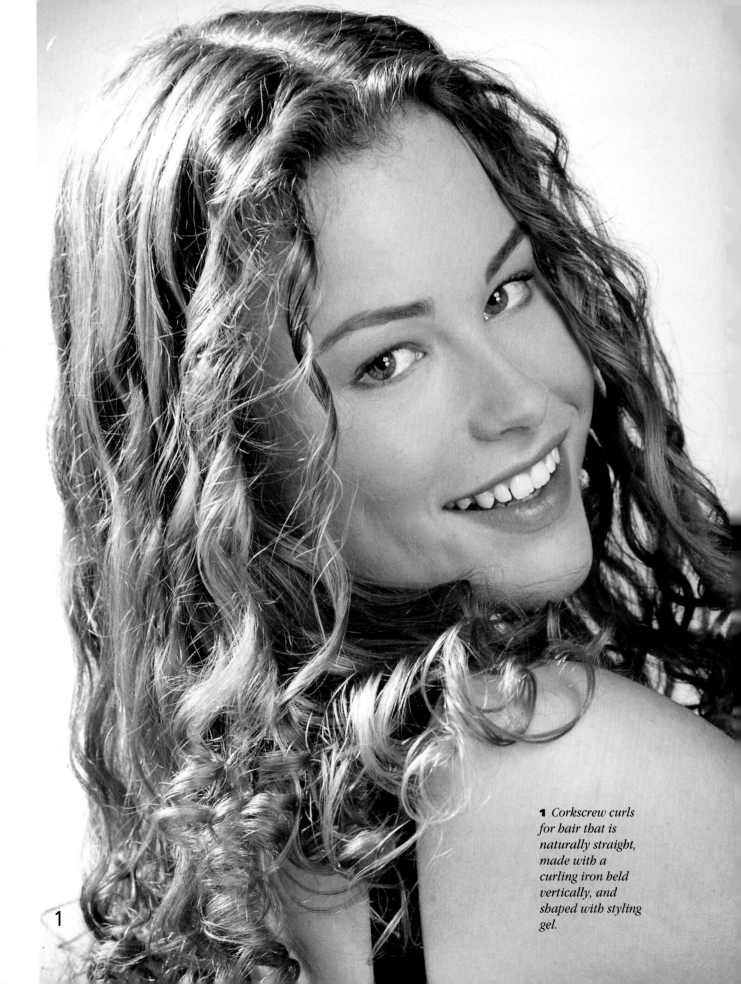

1 *Corkscrew curls for hair that is naturally straight, made with a curling iron held vertically, and shaped with styling gel.*

1

LONG *curly styles*

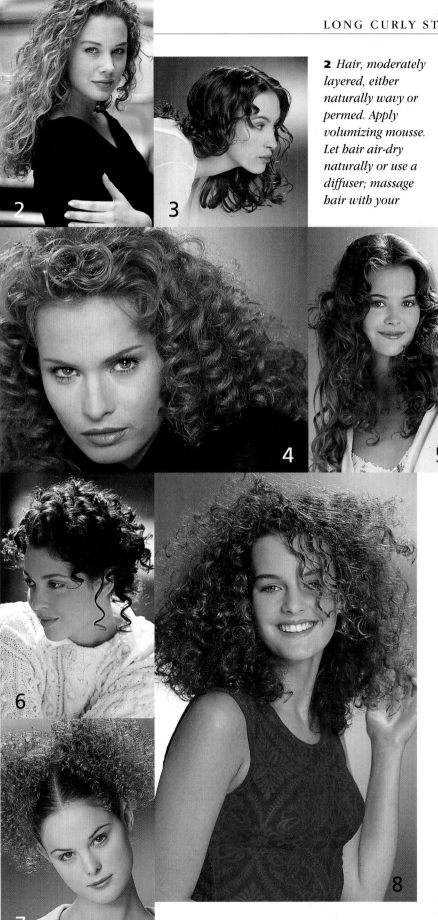

2 *Hair, moderately layered, either naturally wavy or permed. Apply volumizing mousse. Let hair air-dry naturally or use a diffuser; massage hair with your hands. Do not comb.*
3 *Styling gel creates this fashionable wet look for hair that is all one length, either naturally wavy or permed.* **4** *Blunt-cut, unlayered hair is needed for these spiral curls. Dampen with hair lacquer and roll vertically on spiral curlers, one lock at a time. Remove curlers carefully and let curls fall down.*
5 *Straight hair is rolled up on medium-size velvet curlers; when dry, comb out with a wide-tooth comb and shake carefully.*
6 *What appears to be a curly head of short hair is in reality longer than shoulder-length natu-rally wavy hair. Roll the hair up on curlers, but do not comb out; then fasten the locks with side combs or clips.* **8** *Naturally curly hair, shaped into beautiful curls, can be worn in a "natural." It is lightly layered only to the left and right of the part, and the ends are cut frequently all the way around. Massage the hair while blow-drying it with a diffuser; then shake the hair vigorously.*

7 *At the crown, take two small bunches of hair, and shape into small clumps. Attach an Afro-style hairpiece to each clump.*

9 *With a middle part, separate the top layer into thin locks, and braid the locks together to create a ropelike effect. Tie the ends.* **10** *The top layer is loosely tied at the back of the head and shaped into a curly mound, pinned in place. The neck hair falls to the shoulders.* **11** *This is how to tame full, tightly curled natural hair. Massage lots of styling gel into towel-dried hair. Part hair into two waves at the forehead and pull smooth on both sides.* **12** *Part hair in the middle, fasten behind ears. Separate two locks in front, apply styling gel, twist around finger, and let hang down loosely in front.* **13** *Strong natural curls are dried with a diffuser and massaged with styling gel. Pull loosely together in the back and twist a lock of hair around them. Pin in place.* **14** *Hair that is naturally slightly wavy is rolled up on medium-sized curlers. Braid in a very loose french braid (see page 80).*

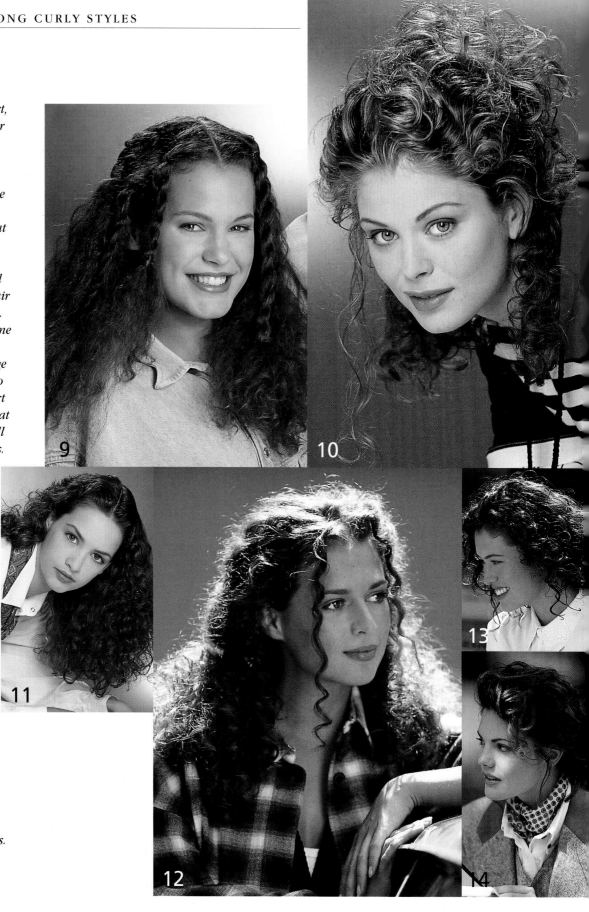

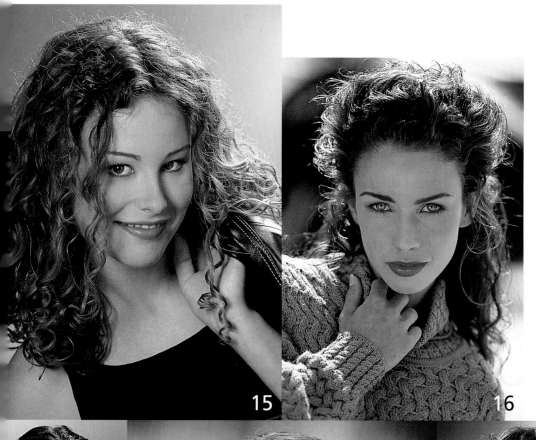

15 *Evenly long, unlayered, naturally wavy hair is rolled on spiral curlers. When hair is dry, apply styling gel and pull it straight a bit.* **16** *Hair is teased well at the forehead and held in place with two large side combs. The back remains loose.* **17** *Waves, following their natural shape, are emphasized with styling gel, a comb, and a brush.* **18** *Corkscrew curls made on straight hair. Spray on setting lotion and roll hair on spiral curlers to ear height. When dry, gather hair together loosely behind the ears with elastics, except for the front lock on each side above the ear, which is held with a small comb.* **19** *Naturally curly hair is made even more curly with curlers. Gather loosely at the neck, turn ends up, and pin in place.* **20** *Spiral curlers can turn bangs and hair at the temples into a veil of curls. Hair at the back is braided.*

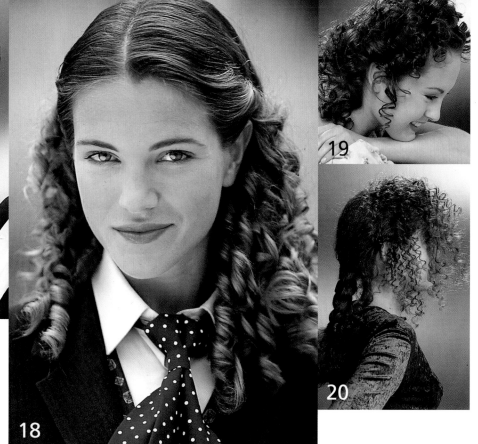

1 *Individual locks of hair are curled with a curling iron. Bend over and tousle hair with fingers. One at a time, gather wide sections and fasten them on top of the head.* **2** *Roll hair on curlers. When dry, tease lightly, pull hair into a ponytail on top of the head, bind with an elastic, and fan out. Brush the ends under.*
4 *Best with naturally wavy hair. Pull the hair up and into a ponytail, bind it with an elastic, and fan out all around. Hair is lightly teased at the roots.*
5 *Tease the top layer at the roots, carefully comb back, and keep it in place with a wide side comb. Pin hair underneath in a small french roll.*
6 *Five knots are made here, tied to look wild on purpose. The ends are sprayed with styling lacquer to make them stick out.* **7** *For medium length, slightly layered hair: tie hair into a ponytail on top of the head, fan out, and separate it into wide locks with the ends turned in and pinned.* **8** *For this super roll, bind hair on top of head in an elastic, twist the elastic, and pull hair halfway through the second loop in the elastic. Pull apart into a wide roll and pin it through the side. The ends in back are left loose.*

3 *Tie hair at the back of the head, twist and pin vertically in a french roll (see pages 78–79).*

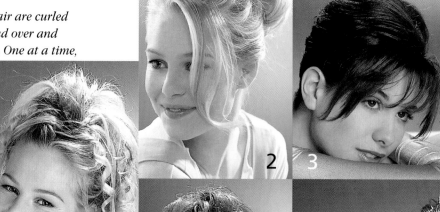

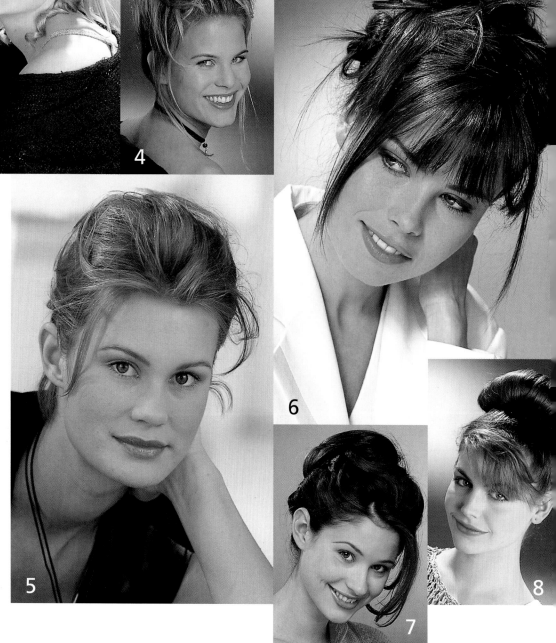

PINNED-UP STYLES *for long hair*

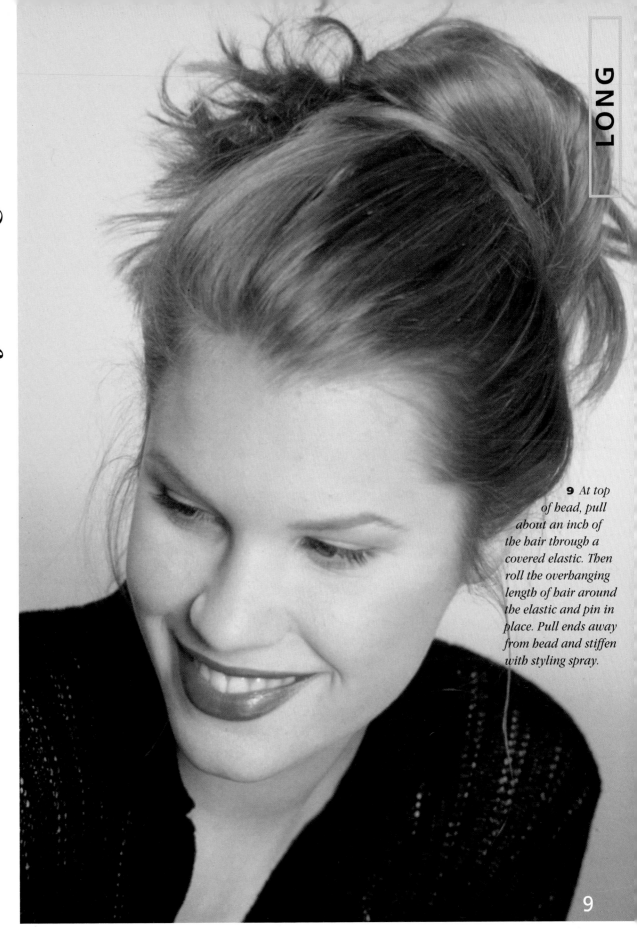

9 *At top of head, pull about an inch of the hair through a covered elastic. Then roll the overhanging length of hair around the elastic and pin in place. Pull ends away from head and stiffen with styling spray.*

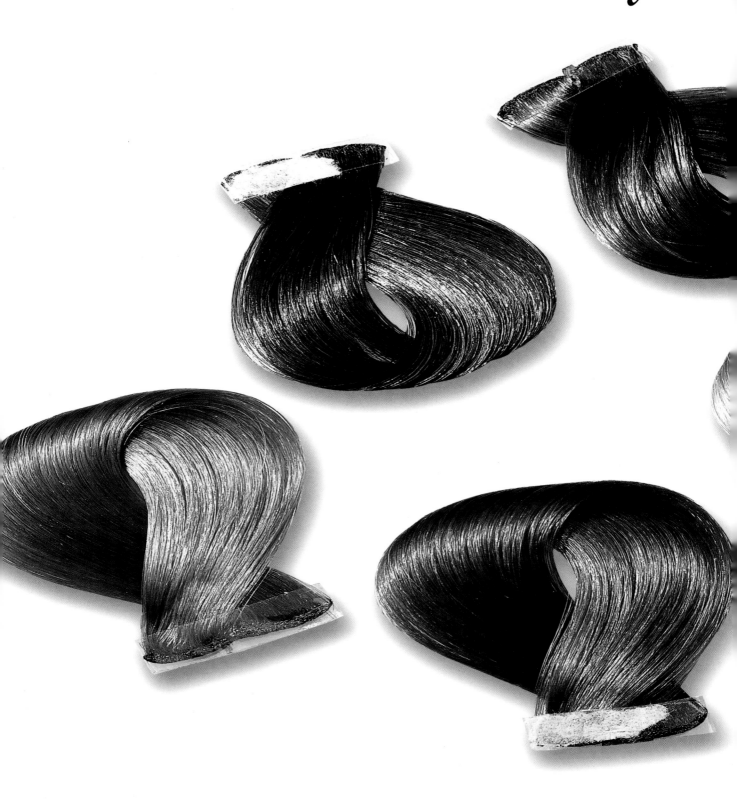

CHAPTER IV

Choose a style

UST FOR YOU

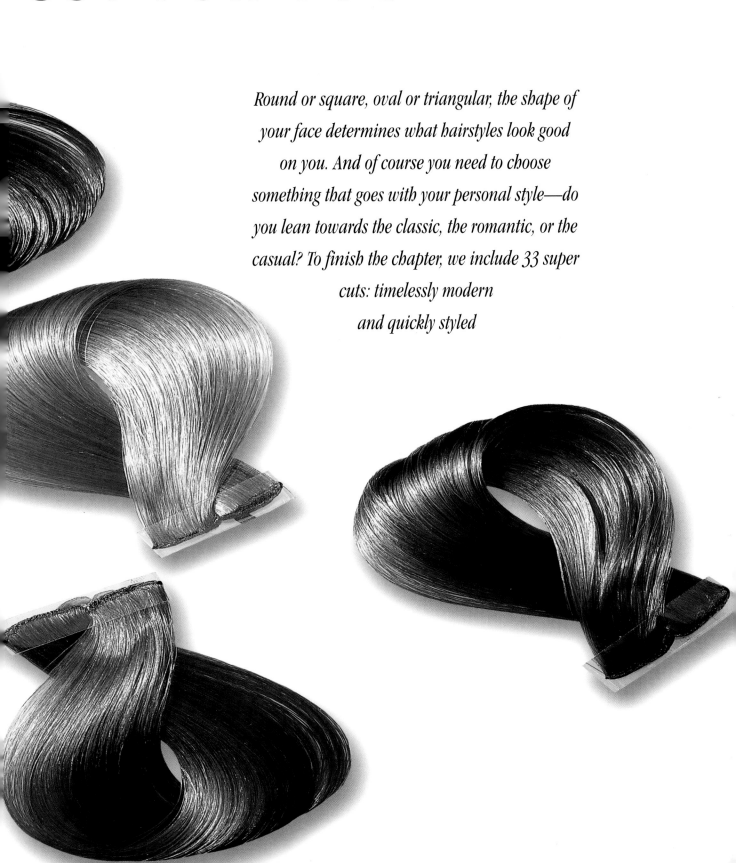

Round or square, oval or triangular, the shape of your face determines what hairstyles look good on you. And of course you need to choose something that goes with your personal style—do you lean towards the classic, the romantic, or the casual? To finish the chapter, we include 33 super cuts: timelessly modern and quickly styled

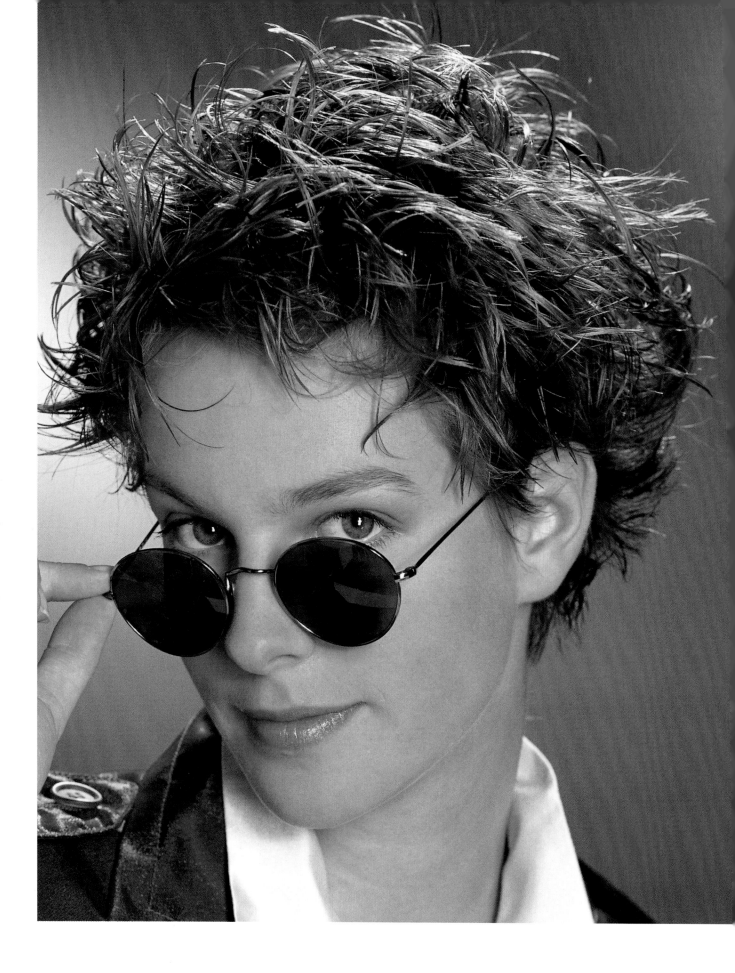

style & FACE SHAPE

This garçon cut with high side part and long side bangs is flattering for every face.

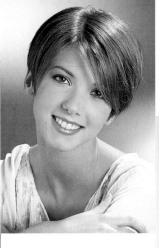

Extremely short hair with long bangs is best for a face that is oval with a high forehead.

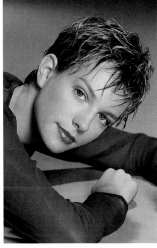

Fullness at the crown is best when a face is elongated and the neck is not too short, because the neck acts as a counterbalance.

A wild and lively mop of curls: a flattering frame for a square or a triangular face with a broad forehead. The curls hang forward in the face.

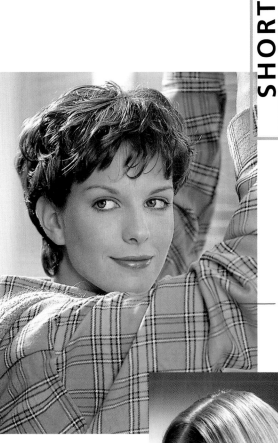

The symbols mean the style is suitable for faces that are

round

oval

square

or triangular

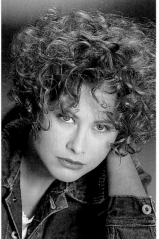

This geometric cut emphasizes the face's triangular shape, instead of concealing it. The chin should not be too pointed.

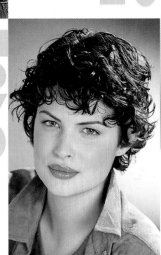

This square-shaped short haircut is a perfect counterbalance to a square chin.

Photo at left:
Such a mop of curls looks best when the shape of the face is oval, but not too elongated.

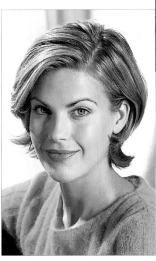

A good frame for every face: Naturally wavy or permed, not too severely layered, and casually tousled with styling gel.

Turned-up ends create an optical counterbalance to a pointed chin.

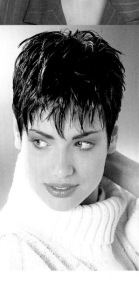

Upturned ends with forehead locks blow-dried to the side create a perfect counterbalance to a pointed chin.

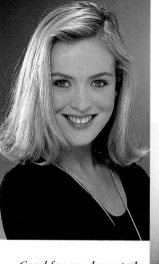

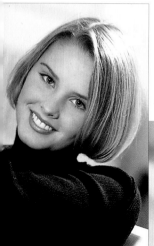

Hair combed close to the head above the forehead, parted in the middle, has ends pulled forward while blow-drying: a good frame for a square or triangular chin.

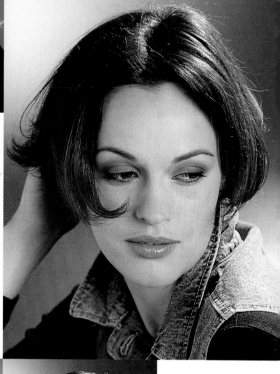

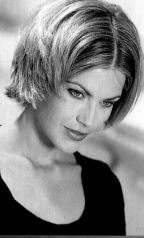

Good for an elongated oval face, but also for a triangular face: a straight bob, blunt-cut at earlobe height.

The higher the side part, the more asymmetrical the hairstyle, and the more becoming for angular faces.

Good for every face shape: a layered bob with full bangs, blow-dried into a round shape; the ends hug the cheeks.

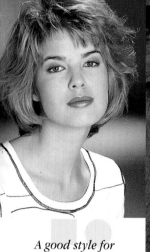

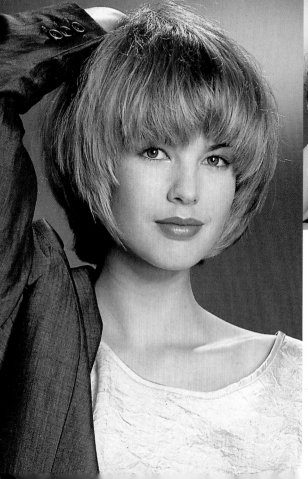

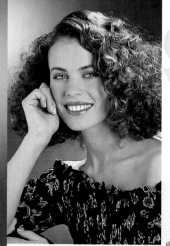

This style creates a full frame, particularly good for very small faces: billowing natural waves or permed, cut slightly below the chin.

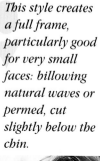

A good style for full cheeks and chin: a feathered bob, with side part, styled in soft tousles.

Good for a narrow face with square or triangular chin: Bob without bangs is blow-dried away from the face.

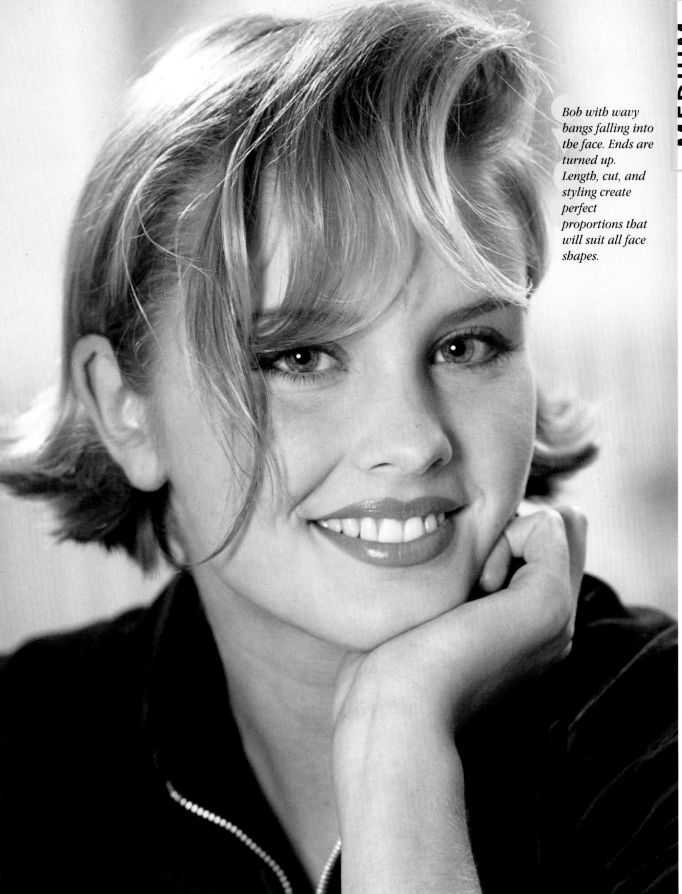

Bob with wavy bangs falling into the face. Ends are turned up. Length, cut, and styling create perfect proportions that will suit all face shapes.

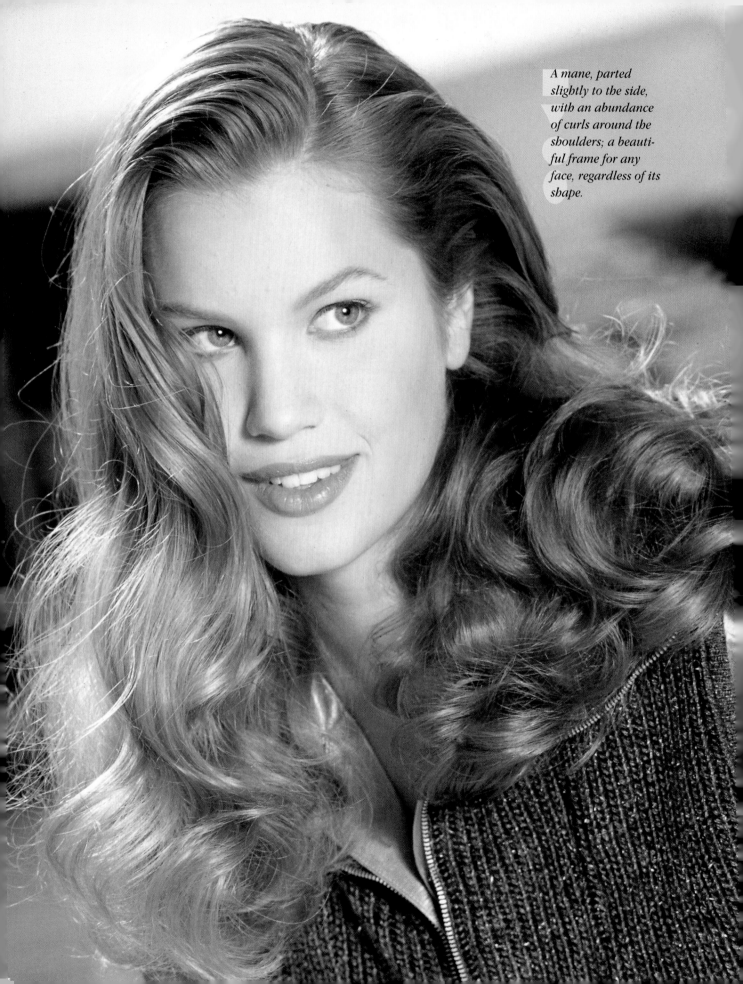

A mane, parted slightly to the side, with an abundance of curls around the shoulders; a beautiful frame for any face, regardless of its shape.

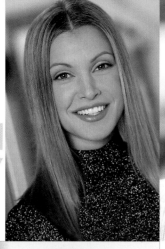

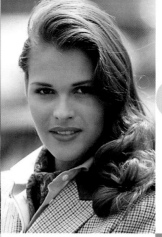

Madonna style, parted in the middle, lengthens a face. Works well with square and triangular chins. The straight, smooth sides are too strong for round faces.

Fullness on one side emphasizes an oval face and looks good when the face is not too narrow.

Cut in layers, ends turned under in blow-drying, with straight full bangs: a perfect frame for a flat face with wide cheekbones.

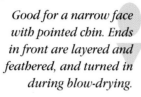

Good for a narrow face with pointed chin. Ends in front are layered and feathered, and turned in during blow-drying.

A flat face with beautiful, clear contour— show it off. A wavy, full style rolled on curlers makes a flattering frame.

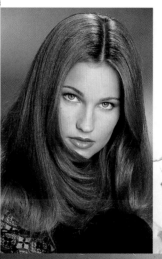

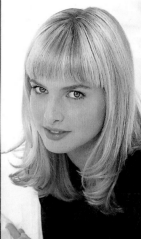

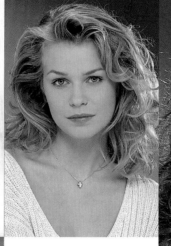

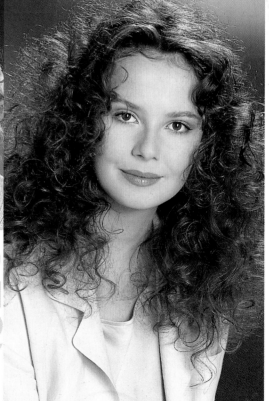

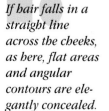

If hair falls in a straight line across the cheeks, as here, flat areas and angular contours are elegantly concealed.

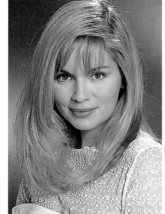

For round faces, this is better than completely straight hair: either naturally wavy or permed, it gently conceals wide cheekbones.

Side part, fringed bangs, and ends softly turned under. Good for all face shapes.

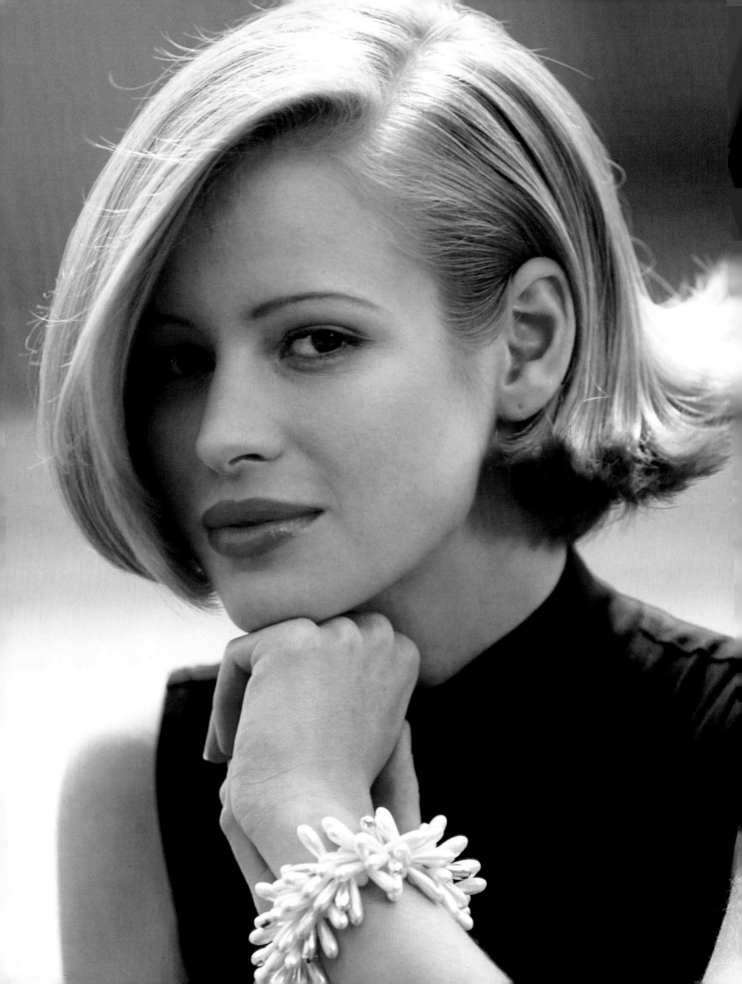

CLASSIC styles

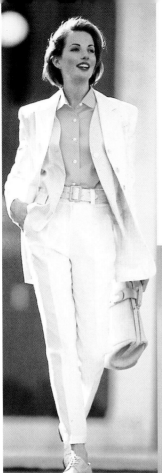

Which style suits you, or which would you like to be? Classic, sporty, romantic? It's great when your personality, clothes, and hairstyle go together

Classic geometric style: short mushroom cut with straight contours from the eyebrows to back behind the ears. Underneath, short at the neck.

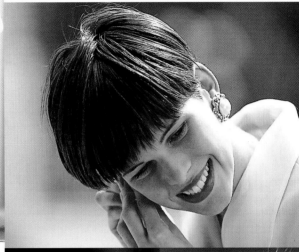

Classic feminine style: long hair worn loose. Roll all hair on large curlers; when dry, carefully brush out.

Elegant and right for every occasion: the classic chin-length bob without bangs. Hair is blow-dried in sections over a round brush and given a touch of styling spray.

Businesslike and feminine: a layered cut with volume in top layer. Brushed back in soft waves and styled over a vent brush.

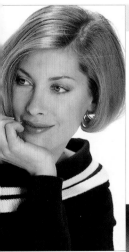

Photo at left:
A classic style with a designer look: Chin-length pageboy without bangs, parted asymmetrically and blow-dried for volume.

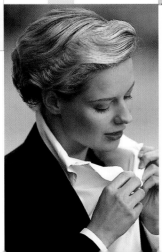

Classic Hollywood: Long hair, accurately parted, with soft waves and ends slightly turned under. Hair is rolled in sections on large rollers; when dry, brush in sections over the back of the hand.

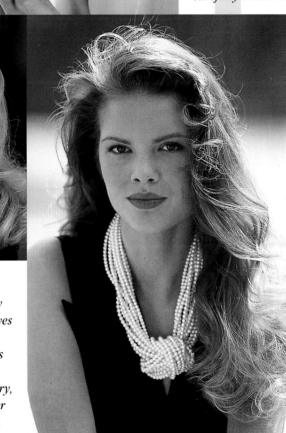

SPORTY *styles*

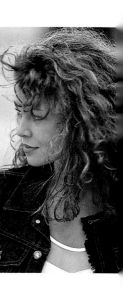

The upturned bangs look as though a gust of wind has blown the hair off the face. With a styling brush, pull hair up, blow-dry, and hold with setting lacquer.

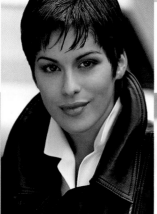

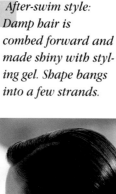

After-swim style: Damp hair is combed forward and made shiny with styling gel. Shape bangs into a few strands.

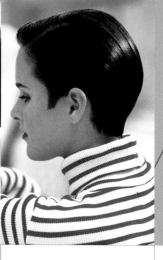

Quickly done after exercising, but also worn for the evening: a layered man's cut, combed close to the head with styling gel.

It doesn't get more casual (and problem-free) than this: Natural curls are cut short and tousled after an application of styling gel.

Casually wild, perfect even under a crash helmet. Naturally wavy hair or a perm, a layered cut, blow-dried with a diffuser and well teased.

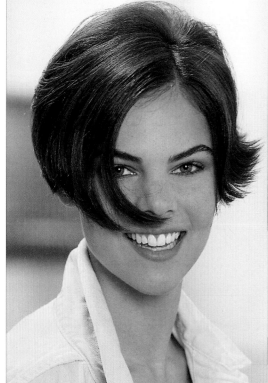

It's the flip at the ends that turns this bob into such a dynamic hairstyle. Pull hair at the roots up from the scalp when blow-drying, and add a little bit of styling spray.

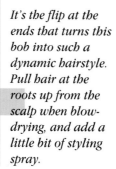

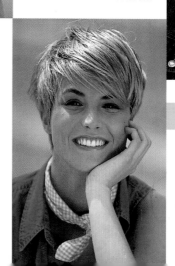

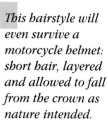

This hairstyle will even survive a motorcycle helmet: short hair, layered and allowed to fall from the crown as nature intended.

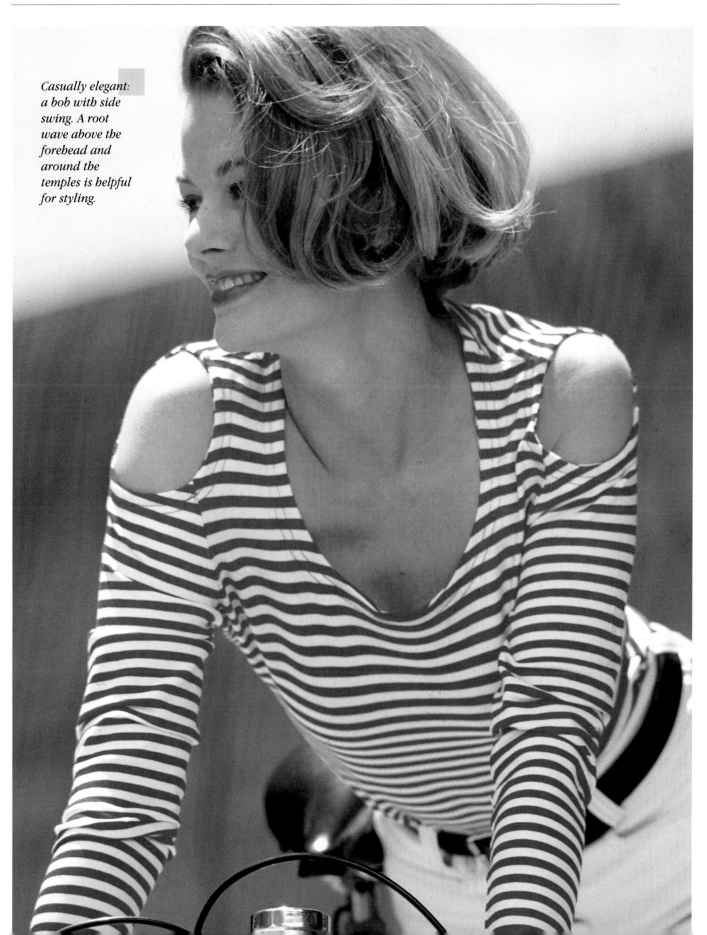

Casually elegant: a bob with side swing. A root wave above the forehead and around the temples is helpful for styling.

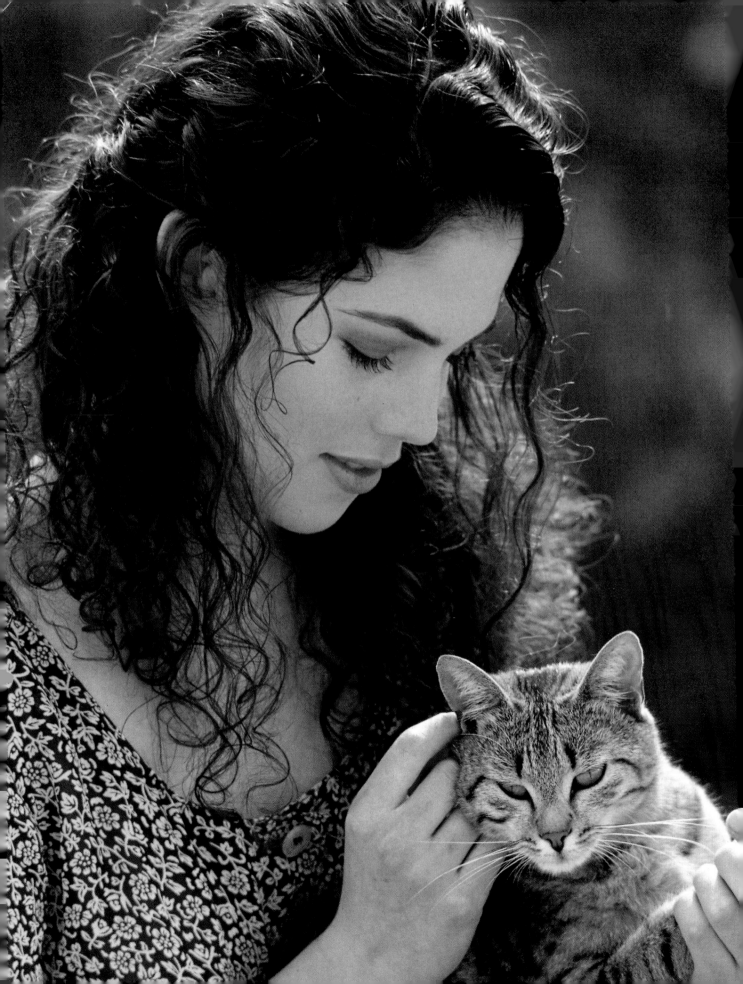

ROMANTIC *styles*

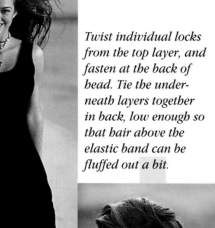

Twist individual locks from the top layer, and fasten at the back of head. Tie the underneath layers together in back, low enough so that hair above the elastic band can be fluffed out a bit.

Tie in a ponytail and roll individual locks on curlers. Pull them apart from each other when hair is dry.

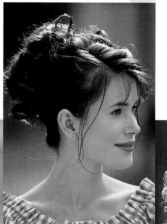

To create these romantic curls, roll hair up on heated curlers. Let cool completely and comb out carefully.

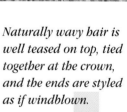

Naturally wavy hair is well teased on top, tied together at the crown, and the ends are styled as if windblown.

Separate the hair at the temples in two sections, and at the back in three sections; then twist the sections around each other, turn up, and secure with a barrette.

Very feminine: long hair with layered contours. After blow-drying, create a wavy look by shaping ends with a curling iron.

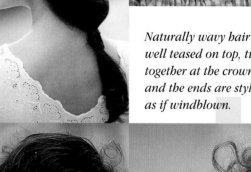

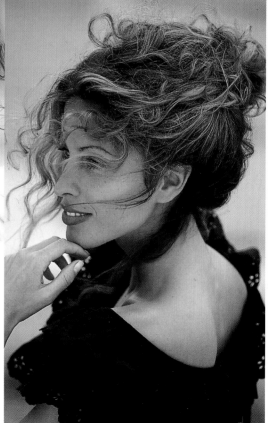

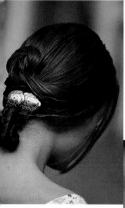

Photo at left: *Purely romantic. Gently tuck hair from around the temples behind ears; strands from above forehead hang loose. Best with naturally wavy hair.*

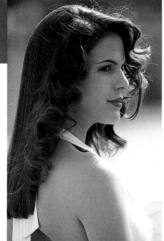

Shoulder-length hair is parted at the back of the head at about ear height in two sections. The upper parts are loosely tied together; the ends are turned under and secured.

SALON APPOINTMENT?

It happens all too often: you leave the hairdresser's and your hair doesn't even come close to what you had in mind. How can that be avoided? What can you do in order to get the hairstyle you want?

Success Strategy 1: Mention that you came on a recommendation

Flattery gets attention, meaning that right from the start, you are not a stranger. It is also good to mention the name of a customer that has frequented the shop for a long time. But how to do all of this, particularly when you are new in town? The easiest way: keep your eyes open at work, on the street, on the bus. Whenever you see a woman with a haircut you like, approach her. She most likely will feel flattered and will be more than willing to provide you with the address of a hairstylist. She may even give you her name. Tell the story to the people at the beauty salon when you go for your appointment.

Success Strategy 2: Choose not only a hairstyle, but also a beauty salon and a hairstylist that fit your personal style

Having the right "chemistry" between you and the hairstylist is as important as his or her professional skills. Do not hesitate to make appointments with different people at the salon you have chosen, until you find the person that's right for you. He or she will be much better able to fulfill your wishes and gain your objectives. You should feel comfortable with your choice. If you need to be relaxed and have the sense that you are cared for, you will not be comfortable with super-modern artists and loud techno music. Then again, if you always need to have the latest style, you might not necessarily want to make an appointment with a "normal" beauty shop; instead, you might choose to go to an "alternative" stylist.

Success Strategy 3: Let them know who you are, particularly by your appearance

The way you dress and use makeup give important clues to the hairstylist about the kind of hairstyle that would appeal to you. Particularly for the first appointment, be sure to choose the kind of clothing that you wear every day—not too dressed up, but also not too casual. If you normally wear a beautiful businesslike hairstyle, don't show up with unstyled unkempt hair at the first appointment with a new hairstylist.

Makeup also is important because it gives you self-confidence, so be sure you are wearing the kind you usually wear. This is very important when you are seated in front of the mirror, shrouded in a hairdresser's cape, with wet hair and a fearful heart.

Five points that speak well for a hairstylist:

1. Your request for a consultation appointment is graciously accepted, even if you don't schedule a cut or styling.
2. The stylist takes time at each appointment for a mini consultation, even before the cape is around your shoulders and your hair is shampooed.
3. The stylist lets you get out of the chair so that you can check your size against your hairstyle. It is important for the proportion between head and body to be correct.
4. The stylist asks about your shampooing and styling habits, e.g., do you shampoo your hair daily, and how much time you have.

SALON APPOINTMENT? DON'T PANIC! **113**

DON'T PANIC!

5. The hairstylist shows you how best to style your haircut and also recommends products that are helpful.

Success Strategy 4: Bring photos or magazines showing styles you like, but be ready to compromise
Examples of hairstyles from magazines or books are a good basis for a discussion during a consultation. But don't insist on any one idea; it might be one that your hair simply is unable to do. Hair that is too short, lacks body, or is in poor health can turn many hairdos into hair don'ts. Should you, however, insist on your ideal, at least be ready to compromise if the hairstylist suggests that, for instance, the damaged ends have to be cut first or the hair has to grow a little longer before you can get what you want.

How well a new haircut turns out, or how good a color or a perm appears, depends in part on how you feel on a given day. That goes for a hairstyle also. Your hormonal cycle has a very distinct influence on how your hair behaves and the condition that it is in. A good or a bad night's sleep is often obvious not only on your face, but also on your hair. Of course, how you will feel on a particular day cannot be predicted exactly. But try to make an appointment that does not fall immediately before or after your menstrual period.

Success Strategy 5: Do not be too radical in your style choice the first time you work with a hairstylist
The first appointment with a new hairstylist and you're immediately trying something radically new? That has all the makings of a disaster! Even a professional must be given the chance to get to know the peculiarities of your hair. He or she needs a chance to observe twice—or maybe even three times—how a particular cut behaves in the course of a month. The same goes for you: only if you are really certain that your hairstylist knows what you like and dislike should you give permission for a radical change like an extremely short haircut or a daring color.

Time your appointments at the hairstylist's properly! A day before an important event—a time when you would like to look your best—is not the ideal time for an appointment. Examples: a job interview, wedding, or a date. You might be very disappointed by the results and consequently depressed—and that influences your appearance. Second, almost every haircut needs a few days so you won't look as if you just walked out of the hairstylist's. A permanent wave also will only look its best after the first week, when the curls have slightly relaxed. For all those reasons, time your salon appointments in such a way that your hair has had time to grow, and so you will have enough time to get comfortable with the results.

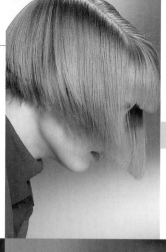

The cut: *Pageboy with precise edges at earlobe height. Slightly layered at the neck. No bangs.* **Styling:** *Apply setting lotion, blow-dry straight with a styling brush, starting at the low side part. Hair on the short side is pulled behind the ear.*

The cut: *Short bob with feathery ends at the height of the mouth.* **Styling:** *Add styling liquid and blow-dry the hair straight over a vent brush, towards the face.*

The cut: *The contours are short and fringed; the front is longer, with a slightly feathery cut. Long wide sideburns are eye-catchers.* **Styling:** *Blow-dry, bending head forward, tousle hair with fingers.*

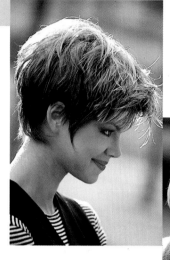

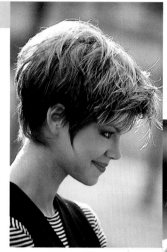

The cut: *Short hair is evenly layered.* **Styling:** *Dampen fingers with styling gel and "comb" hair back with your fingers. Dry with a diffuser.*

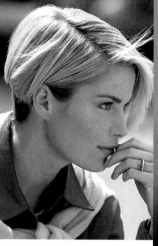

The cut: *Super-short layered cut with fringed contours.* **Styling:** *Apply volumizing mousse, blow-dry opposite the hair's direction of growth. Or let air-dry.*

The cut: *Bob with smooth top layer, triangular at the neck and sides.* **Styling:** *Apply volumizing mousse and blow-dry, creating a rounded look.*

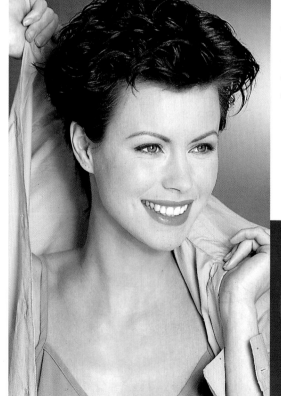

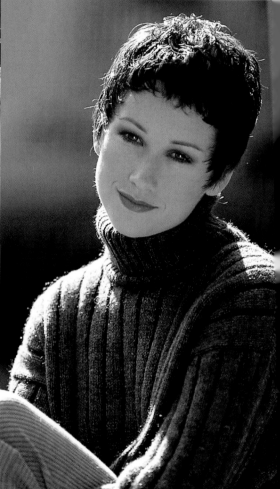

Here it is the cut that makes styling a breeze. It is ideal for people who have very little time in the morning!

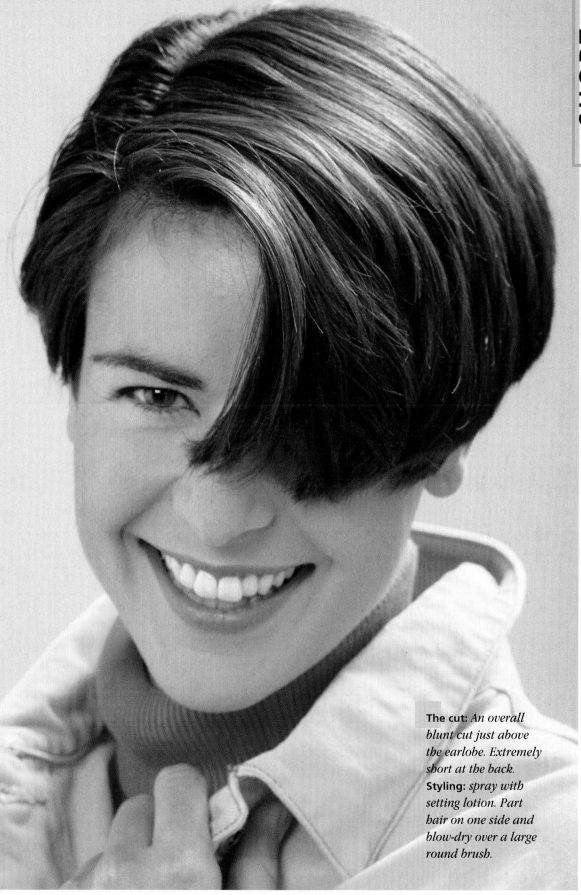

quick-dry **SUPER CUTS**

The cut: *An overall blunt cut just above the earlobe. Extremely short at the back.* **Styling:** *spray with setting lotion. Part hair on one side and blow-dry over a large round brush.*

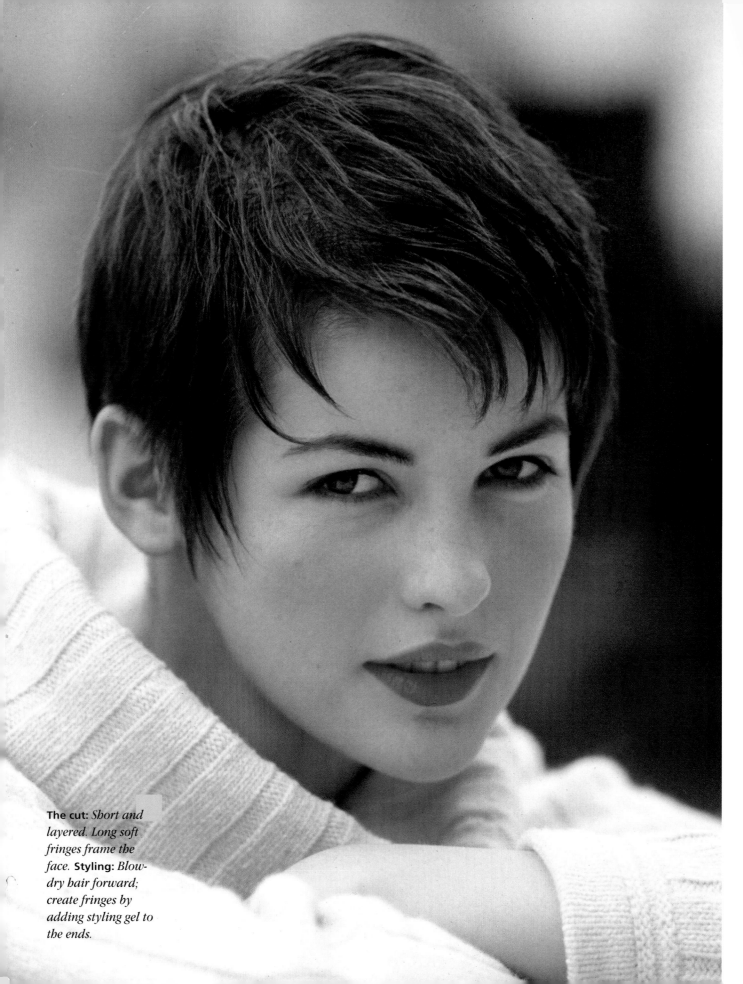

The cut: *Short and layered. Long soft fringes frame the face.* **Styling:** *Blow-dry hair forward; create fringes by adding styling gel to the ends.*

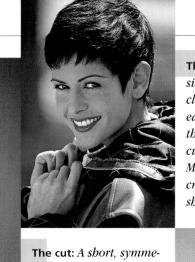

The cut: *Pointed sideburns and a clean cut around the ears are what make this short-layered cut special.* **Styling:** *Move blow-dryer in crisscross pattern; shape and spray.*

The cut: *Hair is cut to one length to the front.* **Styling:** *Blow-dry hair over a vent brush, starting at the crown and working to the forehead. Shape fringes with styling gel.*

The cut: *A short, symmetrical bob with full bangs.* **Styling:** *Dampen hair with styling liquid and blow-dry over a flat brush.*

The cut: *Naturally wavy hair, cut in short layers. At neck, the cut follows the natural hairline.* **Styling:** *Brush hair up when blow-drying.*

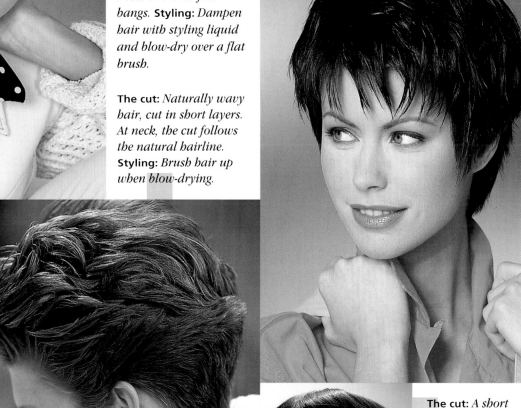

The cut: *Match-stick-length hair, layered with lots of body at the top and extremely short contours.* **Styling:** *Shape with fingers and blow-dry. Apply styling gel in small amounts to the ends.*

The cut: *A short bob with fringes on the side and at the neck.* **Styling:** *Blow-dry all the hair forward over a flat brush. Add a dab of gel wax to the ends and twist them into fringes.*

The cut: *Mushroom cut with long top layer.* **Styling:** *While blow-drying, move spread-out fingers from below through hair; fan out ends.*

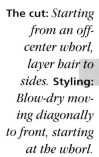

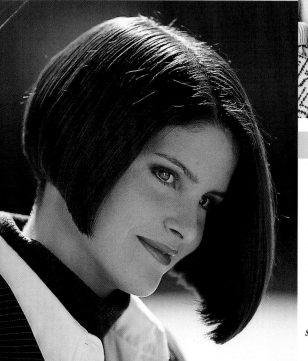

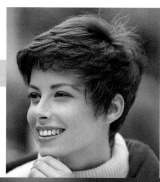

The cut: *Starting from an off-center whorl, layer hair to sides.* **Styling:** *Blow-dry moving diagonally to front, starting at the whorl.*

The cut: *Classic chin-length bob without bangs. The layered neck emphasizes back of head.* **Styling:** *A high part starting at crown; blow-dry over a flat brush, turning in.*

The cut: *The top layer is layered; sideburns are super long; neck hair is short.* **Styling:** *While blow-drying, brush forward.*

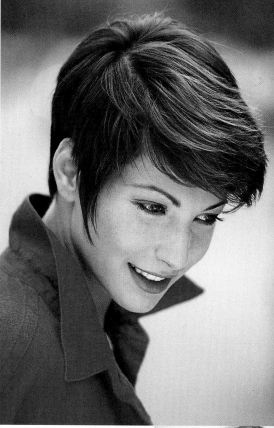

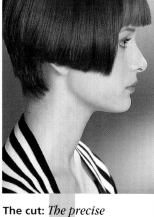

The cut: *The precise edges are evident on this pageboy. The neck hair is layered.* **Styling:** *Add styling lotion and blow-dry everything over a flat brush, pulling the hair down.*

The cut: *An asymmetrical bob without bangs; slightly layered contours.* **Styling:** *With volumizing mousse and a round brush, blow-dry towards the back.*

The cut: *Top layer is almost all one length, hair underneath is thinned out in fringes.* **Styling:** *Blow-dry top layer down over a round brush; turn the underneath layer upwards.*

The cut: *A short bob with long top layer; only the contours are slightly layered.* **Styling:** *Add volumizing mousse and blow-dry over a round brush, pulling brush upwards at the roots.*

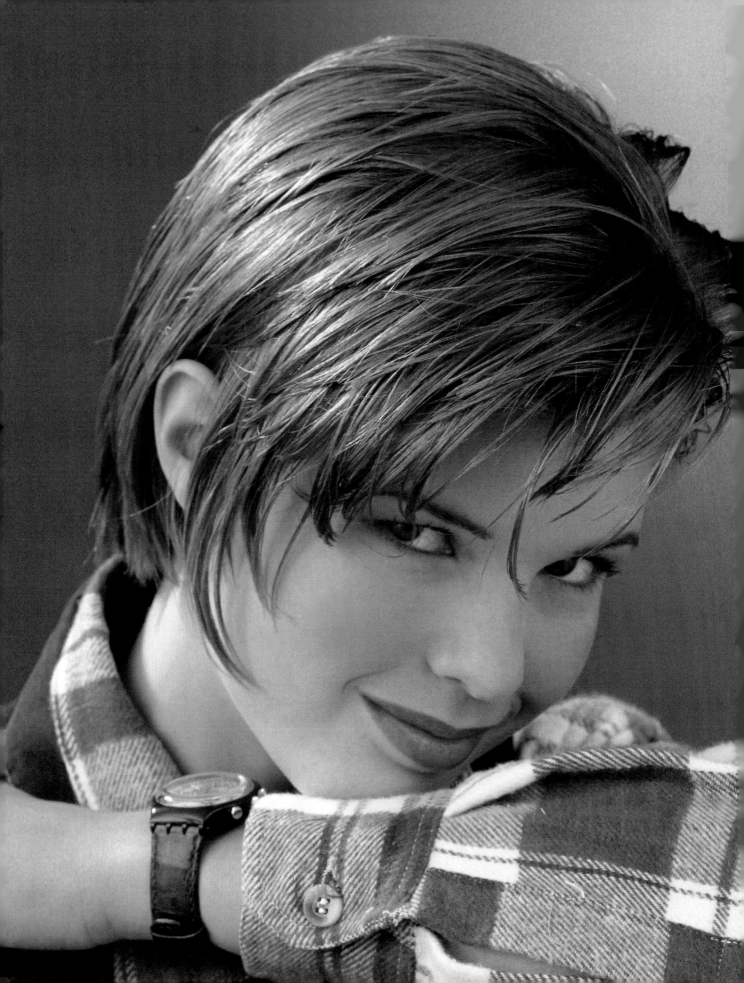

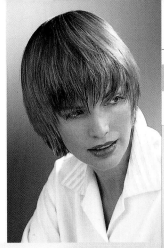

Photo at left: **The cut:** *Front is layered, hair at the neck left full with a blunt cut.* **Styling:** *Blow-dry over a round brush; shape strands by generously applying styling gel.*

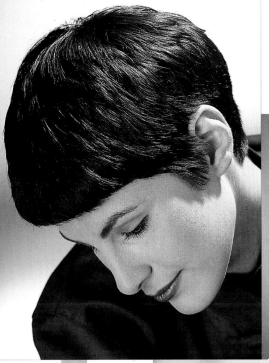

The cut: *A feathery contour, with long top layer.* **Styling:** *Starting at the crown, blow-dry everything forward. The ends around face are fringed with styling gel.*

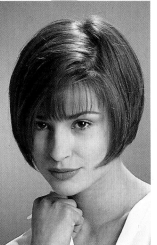

The cut: *A short bob, contoured shorter in back; layered at neck.* **Styling:** *Add a small amount of styling gel, comb smooth, and let air-dry.*

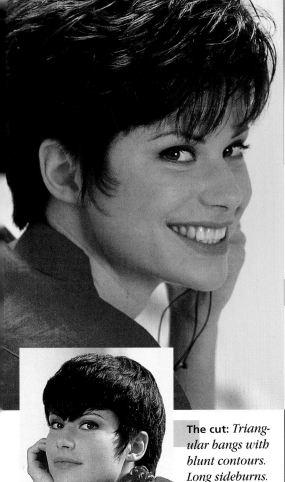

The cut: *Layered cut with helmetlike contour in front.* **Styling:** *With a small amount of styling gel, smooth hair, and let dry naturally.*

The cut: *Short layers in very thick hair; forehead hair and sideburns are fringed.* **Styling:** *While blow-drying, pull the hair up with your fingers and then tousle.*

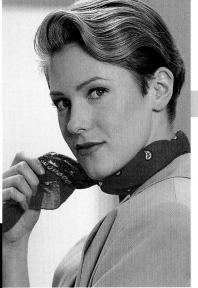

The cut: *Triangular bangs with blunt contours. Long sideburns. In back, everything in short layers.* **Styling:** *Starting at the crown, blow-dry smooth over a brush.*

The cut: *Helmet-cut with heavy bangs and very long sideburns.* **Styling:** *Starting at the crown, blow-dry over a brush, following the cut.*

The cut: *Create smooth waves starting at the forehead. A super-long top layer, with sideburns and short neck hair.* **Styling:** *Massage gel into hair. Comb hair back. Push hair forward with the flat of your hand and let it air-dry naturally.*

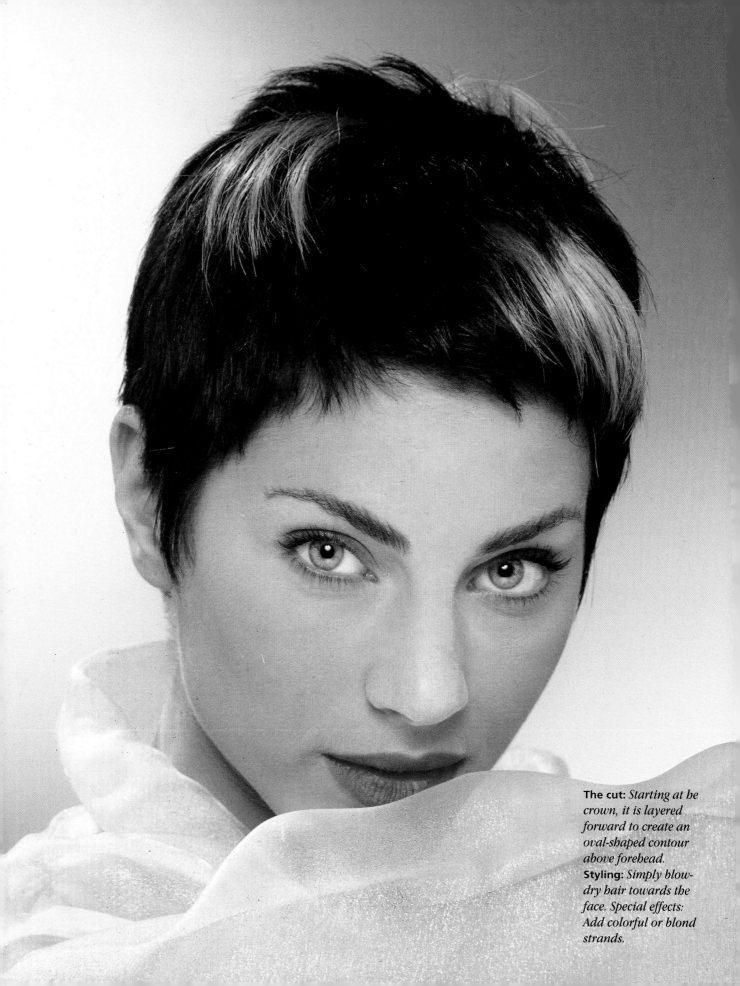

The cut: *Starting at he crown, it is layered forward to create an oval-shaped contour above forehead.*
Styling: *Simply blow-dry hair towards the face. Special effects: Add colorful or blond strands.*

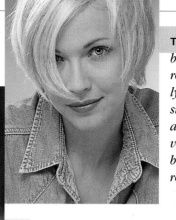

The cut: *Ear-length bob—no bangs. Narrow side is completely layered; the wide side is layered only at ends.* **Styling:** *Add volumizing mousse; blow-dry over a round brush.*

The cut: *Natural curls, layered short at the crown, very long and feathery at the neck.* **Styling:** *Add styling gel, comb back, and let dry naturally.*

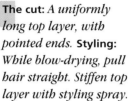

The cut: *A uniformly long top layer, with pointed ends.* **Styling:** *While blow-drying, pull hair straight. Stiffen top layer with styling spray.*

The cut: *A short bob with extreme fringed contours.* **Styling:** *Spray with setting lotion and blow-dry forward.*

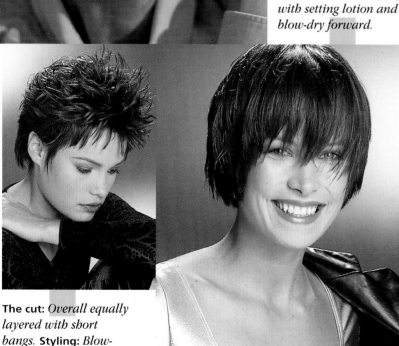

The cut: *Overall equally layered with short bangs.* **Styling:** *Blow-dry, pushing hair back and forth. Add styling gel, pull hair up, and shape into fringes with fingers. A few strands are pulled down over the forehead.*

The cut: *Starting at the back of crown, generously layer the top layer.* **Styling:** *Starting at the crown, blow-dry hair towards the face, using fingers instead of a brush.*

The cut: *Absolutely straight, overall blunt cut. Bangs are cut absolutely straight across.* **Styling:** *With a flat brush, blow-dry smooth; sides are slightly curved forward.*

The cut: *Shoulder-length bob with stylishly fringed contour.* **Styling:** *Blow-dry the sides forward over a round brush, and the neck hair outward. Use styling gel to slightly fringe the ends.*

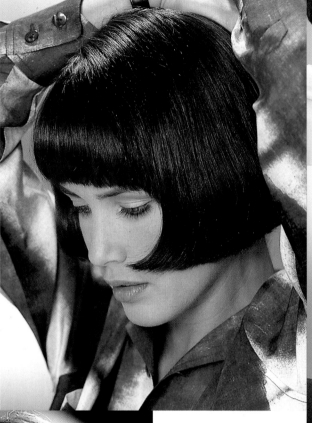

The cut: *The top lay[er] is slightly shorter, making the hair aut[o-] matically move back when you blow-dry [it]. The neck is layered.* **Styling:** *Blow-dry o[n] a round brush towa[rd] the inside.*

The cut: *A pageboy with ends distinctly layered.* **Styling:** *Blow-dry hair over a brush at the roots, and blow-dry the rest outward and forward.*

The cut: *Pageboy of one length, only somewhat shorter at the sides near the face.* **Styling:** *Add volumizing mousse. Bend over and blow-dry hair over a round brush, turning the ends under.*

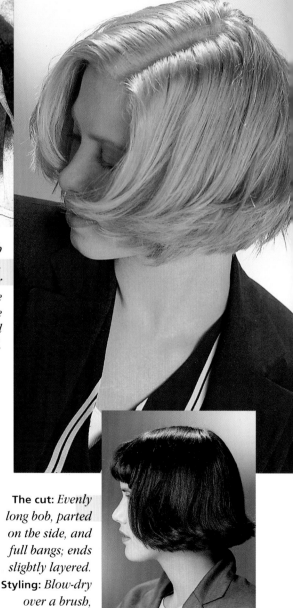

The cut: *Evenly long bob, parted on the side, and full bangs; ends slightly layered.* **Styling:** *Blow-dry over a brush, turning under; turn ends to the back.*

The cut: *Shoulder-length bob, blunt and completely straight all around.* **Styling:** *Add volume to the crown by moving hair dryer across and back. A high but not entirely straight part. Dampen hair roots at forehead and temples with styling gel and blow-dry, lifting hair off the scalp.*

PHOTO CREDITS

Front cover: Peter Pfander. Page 2/3: *freundin-Archiv* magazine. Page 6: Peter Pfander; Hannelore Hopp (4); Tom Biondo; *freundin-Archiv* magazine. Page 7: Peter Pfander (2); Hannelore Hopp (3); Guy Chevalier. Page 8/9: Manfred Spachmann. Page 10/11: Peter Pfander. Page 12: Peter Pfander (3); Guido Bertram. Page 13: Hannelore Hopp. Page 14: Hannelore Hopp (4); Guido Bertram (4). Page 15: Hannelore Hopp (4); Peter Pfander (3). Page 16: Jörg Steffens. Page 17: Jörg Steffens (4); *freundin-Archiv* magazine. Page 18: Tom Biondo (3); Jörg Steffens (3). Page 19: Tom Biondo (5); Jörg Steffens. Page 20/21: Guido Bertram. Page 22/23 Tom Biondo. Page 24/25: Guido Bertram. Page 26 Guido Bertram (4); Hannelore Hopp. Page 27: Hannelore Hopp. Page 28: *freundin-Archiv* magazine. Page 29: Tom Biondo (4); Peter Pfander (4). Page 30: Hannelore Hopp. Page 31: Hannelore Hopp (5); *freundin-Archiv* magazine. Page 32/33: Hannelore Hopp. Page 34/35: Hannelore Hopp. Page 38/39: *freundin-Archiv* magazine. Page 40: Hannelore Hopp. Page 41: Peter Pfander (2); Giovanni Minischetti (2); Olaf Krönke; *freundin-Archiv* magazine. Page 42: Hannelore Hopp (4); Peter Pfander; Olaf Krönke. Page 43: *freundin-Archiv* magazine. Page 44: Hannelore Hopp. Page 45: Guy Chevalier; Guido Bertram; Hannelore Hopp (3). Page 46: Peter Pfander (3); Hannelore Hopp; Gerald Klepka; Ron Nicolaysen. Page 47+48: Peter Pfander. Page 49: Giovanni Minischetti; Olaf Krönke; Tom Biondo; *freundin-Archiv* magazine. Page 50: Ron Nicolaysen; Hannelore Hopp (2); Peter Pfander (2); Olaf Krönke. Page 51: Hannelore Hopp. Page 54 Hannelore Hopp. Page 55: Peter Pfander (4); Hannelore Hopp; Olaf Krönke; *freundin-Archiv* magazine. Page 56: Peter Pfander (2); Hannelore Hopp (4). Page 57: Gerald Klepka. Page 58: Guido Bertram. Page 59: Peter Pfander (3); Otto Rauser; Hannelore Hopp; Gerald Klepka; Olaf Krönke; Tom Biondo. Page 60: Guido Bertram. Page 61: Peter Pfander; Ron Nicolaysen; Guido Bertram; Hannelore Hopp (2); *freundin-Archiv* magazine (2). Page 62: Hannelore Hopp (2); Peter Pfander (2); Giovanni Minischetti. Page 63: Peter Pfander (2); Hannelore Hopp (3). Page 66/67: *freundin-Archiv* magazine. Page 68: Hannelore Hopp. Page 69: Peter Pfander; Hannelore Hopp (3); Giovanni Minischetti (2); *freundin-Archiv* magazine. Page 70: Ron Nicolaysen; Peter Pfander (2); Otto Rauser; Tom Biondo; Olaf Krönke. Page 71: Giovanni Minischetti. Page 72: Hannelore Hopp. Page 73: Hannelore Hopp (2); Peter Pfander (2); Giovanni Minischetti. Page 74: Metta Holst; Peter Pfander (2); Ron Nicolaysen; Gerald Klepka. Page 75: Peter Pfander (3); Guy Chevalier (3). Page 76: Peter Pfander (2); Hannelore Hopp (2); Metta Holst; *freundin-Archiv* magazine (2). Page 77+78: Hannelore Hopp. Page 79: Hannelore Hopp (2); Peter Pfander. Page 80: Giovanni Minischetti; Guy Chevalier. Page 81+82: *freundin-Archiv* magazine. Page 83 Guy Chevalier; *freundin-Archiv* magazine (2). Page 84 Hannelore Hopp. Page 85: *freundin-Archiv* magazine. Page 88: Gerald Klepka. Page 89: Giovanni Minischetti; Peter Pfander (2); Hannelore Hopp (3). Page 90: Peter Pfander (4); Tom Biondo; Hannelore Hopp. Page 91: Otto Rauser. Page 92:

freundin-Archiv magazine. Page 93: Hannelore Hopp (2); Peter Pfander (4); Tom Biondo. Page 94: Peter Pfander (5); Hannelore Hopp. Page 95: Gerald Klepka; Giovanni Mini-schetti (2); Peter Pfander (2). Page 96: Hannelore Hopp (2); Tom Biondo (2); Peter Pfander (3); Guy Chevalier. Page 97: Guido Bertram. Page 98/99: Thomas v. Salomon. Page 100: Peter Pfander. Page 101: Peter Pfander (3); Hannelore Hopp (5). Page 102: Tom Biondo; Hanne-lore Hopp (5); Peter Pfander (2). Page 103+104: Hannelore Hopp; Page 105: Guido Bertram (2); Guy Chevalier; Peter Pfander (3); Tom Biondo; Hanne-lore Hopp. Page 106: *freundin-Archiv* magazine. Page 107: Rafael C. Betzler; Giovanni Minischetti (4); Peter Pfander. Page 108: Olaf Krönke; Hannelore Hopp (3); Giovanni Minischetti (2); Gerald Klepka; Guy Chevalier. Page 109+110: Ron Nicolaysen. Page 111: Ron Nicolaysen (2); Giovanni Minischetti (4); *freundin-Archiv* magazine (2). Page 114: Gerald Klepka; Peter Pfander (3); Hannelore Hopp (2). Page 115: Hannelore Hopp. Page 116: Guy Chevalier. Page 117: Hannelore Hopp; Giovanni Minischetti (2); Peter Pfander (3). Page 118: Peter Pfander (2); Hannelore Hopp (3); Guy Chevalier; *freundin-Archiv* magazine. Page 119+120: Guy Chevalier. Page 121: Guy Chevalier; Hannelore Hopp (2); *freundin-Archiv* magazine; Peter Pfander; Otto Rauser; Giovanni Minischetti. Page 122: Peter Pflander. Page 123: Tom Biondo; Metta Holst; Peter Pfander (2); Hannelore Hopp (2), Page 124; Peter Pfander (2); Hannelore Hopp (2); Giovanni Minischetti; Gerald Klepka. Page 125: Giovanni Minischetti.

INDEX